# METHODS IN MOLECULAR BIOLOGY



*Series Editor*
John M. Walker
School of Life and Medical Sciences
University of Hertfordshire
Hatfield, UK

For further volumes:
http://www.springer.com/series/7651

For over 35 years, biological scientists have come to rely on the research protocols and methodologies in the critically acclaimed *Methods in Molecular Biology* series. The series was the first to introduce the step-by-step protocols approach that has become the standard in all biomedical protocol publishing. Each protocol is provided in readily-reproducible step-by-step fashion, opening with an introductory overview, a list of the materials and reagents needed to complete the experiment, and followed by a detailed procedure that is supported with a helpful notes section offering tips and tricks of the trade as well as troubleshooting advice. These hallmark features were introduced by series editor Dr. John Walker and constitute the key ingredient in each and every volume of the *Methods in Molecular Biology* series. Tested and trusted, comprehensive and reliable, all protocols from the series are indexed in PubMed.

# Adipogenesis

## Methods and Protocols

Edited by

**Michael S. Pepper and Melvin A. Ambele**

*Institute for Cellular and Molecular Medicine, Department of Medical Immunology, and SAMRC Extramural Unit for Stem Cell Research and Therapy, Faculty of Health Sciences, University of Pretoria, Pretoria, South Africa*

Humana Press

*Editors*
Michael S. Pepper
Institute for Cellular and Molecular Medicine, Department of Medical Immunology, and SAMRC Extramural Unit for Stem Cell Research and Therapy, Faculty of Health Sciences
University of Pretoria
Pretoria, South Africa

Melvin A. Ambele
Institute for Cellular and Molecular Medicine, Department of Medical Immunology, and SAMRC Extramural Unit for Stem Cell Research and Therapy, Faculty of Health Sciences
University of Pretoria
Pretoria, South Africa

ISSN 1064-3745 ISSN 1940-6029 (electronic)
Methods in Molecular Biology
ISBN 978-1-0716-4609-0 ISBN 978-1-0716-4607-6 (eBook)
https://doi.org/10.1007/978-1-0716-4607-6



This Humana imprint is published by the registered company Springer Science+Business Media, LLC, part of Springer Nature.
The registered company address is: 1 New York Plaza, New York, NY 10004, U.S.A.

# Preface

The field of molecular cell biology is advancing rapidly, as the complexity of biological processes is progressively unraveled. As the granularity increases, so do the opportunities to translate research findings into clinically relevant applications. Adipogenesis is at the heart of obesity, which is one of the major contributors to morbidity and mortality across the world. Studying adipogenesis is therefore highly relevant and has borne fruit in terms of broadening the knowledge base and clinical applications.

This book is a compilation of methods and protocols that are currently being used to explore adipogenesis from cellular and molecular perspectives, and which have contributed significantly to the body of knowledge in the field. The chapters are contributed by senior postgraduate students with practical, hands-on experience and expertise in specific methods and protocols, as well as by senior researchers who are leading experts in the field.

Novel molecular players and mechanisms continue to be uncovered in the adipogenesis field, although knowledge on the roles of both known and novel molecular factors in this complex, multistep process of adipogenesis, remains limited. This book is intended for researchers, students, and other stakeholders in the field of adipogenesis. Each chapter provides practical step-by-step details for hands-on experimentation, ensuring a high level of reproducibility in data quality, which is essential for the advancement of knowledge in the field.

We would like to thank all the contributing authors for sharing detailed accounts of their well-optimized, in-house day-to-day practical methods and protocols in adipogenesis research, without which this book would not have been possible. We also extend our gratitude to the Institute for Cellular and Molecular Medicine and the SAMRC Extramural Unit for Stem Cell Research and Therapy, University of Pretoria, South Africa, for providing some of the resources needed for the preparation, editing, and finalization of this book. In preparing this book we had to draw on our collective experience in studying adipogenesis, which was funded by the entities mentioned above.

*Pretoria, South Africa*

*Michael S. Pepper*
*Melvin A. Ambele*

# Contents

# Contributors

LADISLAUS TAPIWA ADAM • *Institute for Cellular and Molecular Medicine, Department of Medical Immunology, and SAMRC Extramural Unit for Stem Cell Research and Therapy, Faculty of Health Sciences, University of Pretoria, Pretoria, South Africa*

MELVIN A. AMBELE • *Institute for Cellular and Molecular Medicine, Department of Medical Immunology, and SAMRC Extramural Unit for Stem Cell Research and Therapy, Faculty of Health Sciences, University of Pretoria, Pretoria, South Africa*

MIGUEL ANGEL • *Departamento de Biología Celular y Fisiología, Instituto de Investigaciones Biomédicas, Universidad Nacional Autónoma de México, Mexico City, Mexico*

ANASTASIOS ATHANASIADIS • *Institute for Cellular and Molecular Medicine, Department of Medical Immunology, and SAMRC Extramural Unit for Stem Cell Research and Therapy, Faculty of Health Sciences, University of Pretoria, Pretoria, South Africa*

CARINA C. BABBO • *Institute for Cellular and Molecular Medicine, Department of Medical Immunology, and SAMRC Extramural Unit for Stem Cell Research and Therapy, Faculty of Health Sciences, University of Pretoria, Pretoria, South Africa*

LISA MARIE BOSMAN • *Institute for Cellular and Molecular Medicine, Department of Medical Immunology, and SAMRC Extramural Unit for Stem Cell Research and Therapy, Faculty of Health Sciences, University of Pretoria, Pretoria, South Africa*

EMILY CRESSWELL • *Oxford Centre for Diabetes, Endocrinology and Metabolism University of Oxford, Churchill Hospital, Oxford, UK*

JAMIE DE BEER • *Institute for Cellular and Molecular Medicine, Department of Medical Immunology, and SAMRC Extramural Unit for Stem Cell Research and Therapy, Faculty of Health Sciences, University of Pretoria, Pretoria, South Africa*

XIMENA DEL TORO-RIOS • *Departamento de Biología Celular y Fisiología, Instituto de Investigaciones Biomédicas, Universidad Nacional Autónoma de México, Mexico City, Mexico*

CHRISNA DURANDT • *Institute for Cellular and Molecular Medicine, Department of Medical Immunology, and SAMRC Extramural Unit for Stem Cell Research and Therapy, Faculty of Health Sciences, University of Pretoria, Pretoria, South Africa*

SANCHEZ RAMIREZ EDGAR • *Departamento de Biología Celular y Fisiología, Instituto de Investigaciones Biomédicas, Universidad Nacional Autónoma de México, Mexico City, Mexico*

JONATHAN M. GAMWELL • *Oxford Centre for Diabetes, Endocrinology and Metabolism University of Oxford, Churchill Hospital, Oxford, UK*

RACHEL GILES • *Institute for Cellular and Molecular Medicine, Department of Medical Immunology, and SAMRC Extramural Unit for Stem Cell Research and Therapy, Faculty of Health Sciences, University of Pretoria, Pretoria, South Africa*

MURRAY GLEN LOGAN • *Institute for Cellular and Molecular Medicine, Department of Medical Immunology, and SAMRC Extramural Unit for Stem Cell Research and Therapy, Faculty of Health Sciences, University of Pretoria, Pretoria, Gauteng, South Africa*

LORENA AGUILAR-ARNAL • *Departamento de Biología Celular y Fisiología, Instituto de Investigaciones Biomédicas, Universidad Nacional Autónoma de México, Mexico City, Mexico*

Alex Leah Marais • *Institute for Cellular and Molecular Medicine, Department of Medical Immunology, and SAMRC Extramural Unit for Stem Cell Research and Therapy, Faculty of Health Sciences, University of Pretoria, Pretoria, Gauteng, South Africa*
Juanita Mellet • *Institute for Cellular and Molecular Medicine, Department of Medical Immunology, and SAMRC Extramural Unit for Stem Cell Research and Therapy, Faculty of Health Sciences, University of Pretoria, Pretoria, Gauteng, South Africa*
Pontsho Moela • *Division of Genetics, Faculty of Natural and Agricultural Sciences, Department of Biochemistry, Genetics, and Microbiology, University of Pretoria, Pretoria, South Africa; Division of Genetics, Department of Biochemistry, Genetics, and Microbiology, Forestry and Agricultural Biotechnology Institute, Faculty of Natural and Agricultural Sciences, University of Pretoria, Pretoria, South Africa*
Thabiso Eric Motaung • *Faculty of Natural and Agricultural Sciences, Department of Biochemistry, Genetics, and Microbiology, Forestry and Agricultural Biotechnology Institute, University of Pretoria, Pretoria, South Africa*
Lilia G. Noriega • *Departamento de Fisiología de la Nutrición, Instituto Nacional de Ciencias Médicas y Nutrición Salvador Zubirán, Mexico City, Mexico*
Olmedo-Suarez • *Departamento de Biología Celular y Fisiología, Instituto de Investigaciones Biomédicas, Universidad Nacional Autónoma de México, Mexico City, Mexico*
Michael S. Pepper • *Institute for Cellular and Molecular Medicine, Department of Medical Immunology, and SAMRC Extramural Unit for Stem Cell Research and Therapy, Faculty of Health Sciences, University of Pretoria, Pretoria, South Africa*
Kimberly Thando Peta • *Institute for Cellular and Molecular Medicine, Department of Medical Immunology, and SAMRC Extramural Unit for Stem Cell Research and Therapy, Faculty of Health Sciences, University of Pretoria, Pretoria, South Africa*
Katherine E. Pinnick • *Oxford Centre for Diabetes, Endocrinology and Metabolism University of Oxford, Churchill Hospital, Oxford, UK*
Reabetswe R. Pitere • *Institute for Cellular and Molecular Medicine, Department of Medical Immunology, and SAMRC Extramural Unit for Stem Cell Research and Therapy, Faculty of Health Sciences, University of Pretoria, Pretoria, South Africa*

# Chapter 1

# Adipogenic Differentiation from Human Embryonic Stem Cells Through Formation of Embryoid Bodies

**Miguel Angel Olmedo-Suárez, Edgar Sánchez-Ramírez, and Lorena Aguilar-Arnal**

## Abstract

In the context of adipogenesis, new adipocytes arise from the differentiation of pluripotent stem cells, including embryonic stem cells (hESCs). This process involves two fundamental phases: lineage commitment and terminal differentiation. This chapter elucidates a comprehensive 22-day protocol designed for the differentiation of the hESC cell line H9 toward the adipogenic lineage.

During the initial phase, we initiate the differentiation process by forming embryoid bodies (EBs). This is achieved by culturing hESCs in an ultralow attachment plate for a duration of 12 days, during which the EBs are exposed to retinoic acid (RA) for a period of 3 days. Subsequently, adipocyte induction is facilitated by transferring EBs onto Geltrex-coated 6-well plates and subjecting them to adipogenic differentiation medium for an additional 10 days. To assess the successful internalization of lipids within the adipocytes, we employ Oil Red O staining. This protocol provides a robust framework for studying adipogenesis from pluripotent stem cells, offering insights into the intricate process of adipocyte development and serving as a valuable tool for related research endeavors.

**Key words** Human embryonic stem cells Adipogenic differentiation, Embryoid bodies, Adipogenesis

## 1 Introduction

Adipose tissue, a metabolically dynamic organ primarily composed of adipocytes, plays a pivotal role in the regulation of metabolism and lipid homeostasis and serves as the primary reservoir for energy storage [1, 2]. Adipogenesis, the process by which new adipocytes form, involves the differentiation of mesenchymal stem cells (MSCs) and, in some cases, pluripotent stem cells, such as embryonic stem cells (ESCs), and induced pluripotent stem cells (iPSCs). This intricate process is orchestrated by a tightly coordinated sequence of gene expression programs and metabolic transitions

Authors Miguel Angel Olmedo-Suárez and Edgar Sánchez Ramírez have equally contributed to this chapter.

Michael S. Pepper and Melvin A. Ambele (eds.), *Adipogenesis: Methods and Protocols*, Methods in Molecular Biology, vol. 2938, https://doi.org/10.1007/978-1-0716-4607-6_1,

[3, 4]. Developing innovative techniques for differentiating human pluripotent stem cells into adipocytes holds the potential to provide profound insights into the mechanisms of adipogenesis and metabolic alterations associated with health and disease and paves the way toward specialized stem cell therapies and regenerative medicine approaches [5].

The differentiation journey from human embryonic stem cells (hESC) to adipocytes can be delineated into two main phases: lineage commitment and terminal differentiation [4]. During the commitment phase, stem cells commit to becoming preadipocytes [4]. To replicate the in vivo environment more faithfully during this phase, a model involving the formation of embryoid bodies (EBs) has been adopted. EBs, which are three-dimensional aggregates, not only give rise to germ layer derivatives but also mimic the earliest stages of embryonic development [6]. In the subsequent phase, the preadipocytes progressively acquire the characteristics of mature adipocytes, including specific physiological functions such as lipid synthesis, insulin sensitivity, and secretion of adipocyte-specific proteins [4, 7].

Here, we describe a protocol for differentiating a hESC cell line toward the adipogenic lineage (Fig. 1) [8]. The differentiation process unfolds in two key phases. In the initial phase, we generate embryoid bodies (EBs) within ultralow attachment well plates and treat them with EB culture medium enriched with retinoic acid (RA). RA, an essential vitamin, not only plays a critical role in early embryoid body formation and development [9], but also regulates germ layer formation [10]. Moreover, it promotes adipocyte differentiation, facilitates fatty acid transport, and contributes to triacylglycerol synthesis [11, 12]. Finally, these EBs are transferred

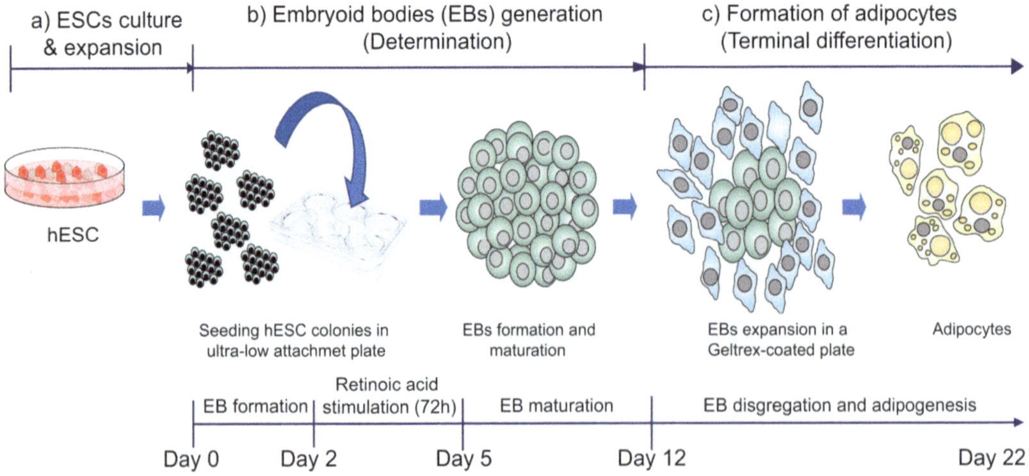


**Fig. 1** Schematic diagram of the experimental procedure. The differentiation method consists of three main steps: stem cell culture and expansion; embryoid body formation and maturation, and terminal adipogenesis

onto Geltrex-coated 6-well plates, where they continue differentiating in adipogenic differentiation medium for an additional 10 days, ultimately culminating in terminal differentiation.

## 2 Materials

Plasticware and liquids used for cell culture must be sterile. All reagents should be stored at 4 °C, and it should be brought to room temperature before using them on cells unless otherwise specified. Avoid heating reagents and media. When using reagents stored at −20 °C, avoid repeated freeze–thaw cycles by aliquoting the reagents into smaller volumes. All solutions must be prepared using ultrapure water and analytical-grade reagents.

### 2.1 Stem Cell Culture

1. Human embryonic stem cell line H9 (WA09, WiCell Research Institute, Inc.).
2. mTeSR Plus medium (STEMCELL Technologies).
3. Penicillin–streptomycin solution.
4. 6-well tissue culture plates.
5. Cell scrapers.
6. DMEM/F-12.
7. HEPES.
8. KnockOut™ Serum Replacement.
9. MEM Non-Essential Amino Acids Solution.
10. L-Glutamine.
11. Geltrex™ LDEV-Free Reduced Growth Factor Basement Membrane (*see* **Note 1**).
12. 2-Mercaptoethanol.
13. Rho kinase inhibitor (iROCK): Prepare an iROCK stock solution of 10 mM in DMSO. Add mTeSR medium to 10 μM.
14. Dulbecco's Phosphate Buffered Saline.
15. Retinoic acid.
16. Dispase (1 U/mL).
17. 37 °C cell culture incubator (37 °C/5% $CO_2$/95% air).
18. Centrifuge.
19. Laminar flow hood.
20. Inverted microscope connected to a camera.

### 2.2 Generation of Embryoid Bodies in Ultralow Attachment Plates

1. Embryoid body medium (EB medium): Prepare the EB medium by mixing the following components: 80% of DMEM/F-12, HEPES, 20% of KnockOut™ Serum Replacement, 1× MEM Non-Essential Amino Acids Solution, 1 mM L-glutamine, 0.1 mM 2-mercaptoethanol (*see* **Note 2**), and 1× penicillin–streptomycin. After mixing all the components, the ESC medium should be filtered using a 0.22 μM filter and stored at 4 °C for approximately 1 month.
2. EB medium supplemented with retinoic acid (EB-RA): Supplement retinoic acid to the EB medium at a final concentration of 100 nM (*see* **Note 3**).
3. A 70 μm cell strainer, sterile.
4. Ultralow attachment 6-well plate with lid and flat bottom.

### 2.3 Adipogenic Differentiation and Lipid Staining

1. Adipogenic differentiation media: MesenCult Adipogenic Differentiation Kit medium.
2. Oil Red O (ORO) stock solution: Weigh out 625 mg of ORO reagent (Sigma-Aldrich O025-25G), and add in 100 mL of isopropyl alcohol. Mix the solution by stirring for 2 h at room temperature, RT (20–25 °C). The solution can be stored at RT for up to 3 months.
3. 4% paraformaldehyde (PFA) in PBS.
4. 60% isopropanol solution in sterile water.

## 3 Methods

Carry out all the procedures at room temperature under sterile conditions unless otherwise specified.

### 3.1 hESC Cell Line Culture and Maintenance

1. Thaw an aliquot of 100 μL of Geltrex on ice (*see* **Note 1**), and immediately add 10 mL of DMEM/F12 medium, and mix the solution.
2. Distribute 1.5 mL of the Geltrex–DMEM/F12 solution to each well in a 6-well plate.
3. Place the 6-well plate inside the cell culture incubator for at least 2 h prior to seeding the cells.
4. Remove carefully the Geltrex–DMEM/F12 solution from the well using a pipette, and immediately add 1 mL of mTeSR Plus supplemented with 10 μM of iROCK (mTeSR–iROCK) to avoid drying of the well before seeding the cells.
5. Thaw a hESC cryovial with approximately one million cells in a water bath at 37 °C. Then, immediately transfer the cell suspension to a conical tube with 5 mL of mTeSR Plus medium.

6. Centrifuge at 800× *g* for 4 min at RT.
7. Remove the supernatant, and add 1 mL of mTeSR–iROCK to resuspend the cell pellet.
8. Transfer the cell suspension into two Geltrex-conditioned wells with the mTeSR–iROCK medium, and shake gently to evenly distribute the colonies.
9. Incubate the plate for 24 h at 37 °C, 5% $CO_2$.
10. Replace the mTeSR–iROCK with 2 mL of mTeSR medium without iROCK.
11. When hESC colonies reach 30% confluence, the mTeSR medium should be replaced daily to maintain hESC in a pluripotent state.
12. When hESC colonies reach 70 or 80% confluence (approximately 4–6 days after seeding), and no signs of differentiation are seen, proceed with the embryoid bodies generation protocol.

### 3.2 Embryoid Bodies (EBs) Generation and Adipogenic Differentiation

To generate embryoid bodies and subsequent adipogenic differentiation, a 22-day differentiation protocol is followed, as shown in Fig. 1.

1. Wash the cells within the plate with 2 mL of DMEM/F12 (without serum).
2. Dissociate the colonies by adding 1 mL of Dispase to each well.
3. Incubate the plate for 7–8 min at 37 °C.
4. Discard the Dispase solution, and wash the cells with 1 mL of DMEM/F12 using a pipette.
5. Add 1 mL of EB medium, and carefully detach the colonies using a cell scraper (Fig. 2a) (*see* **Note 4**).
6. Use a pipette to collect the hESC colonies suspended in EB medium, and take a 70 μm cell strainer (Fig. 2b), and transfer the cell suspension to the top of the cell strainer (Fig. 2c) (*see* **Note 5**).
7. Collect the remaining colonies in the plate with 1 mL of EB medium, and pass through the cell strainer.
8. Wash the colonies in the filter twice with 1 mL of DMEM/F12.
9. Invert the cell strainer into a well of an ultralow attachment plate, and add 1 mL of EB–iROCK medium, or as needed to pull colonies out of the cell strainer and into the well (Fig. 2d).
10. Distribute hESC colonies in EB–iROCK medium homogeneously within three ultralow attachment wells, leaving a volume of about 1 mL of EB–iROCK medium in each well.
11. Shake the plate gently and incubate it at 37 °C.

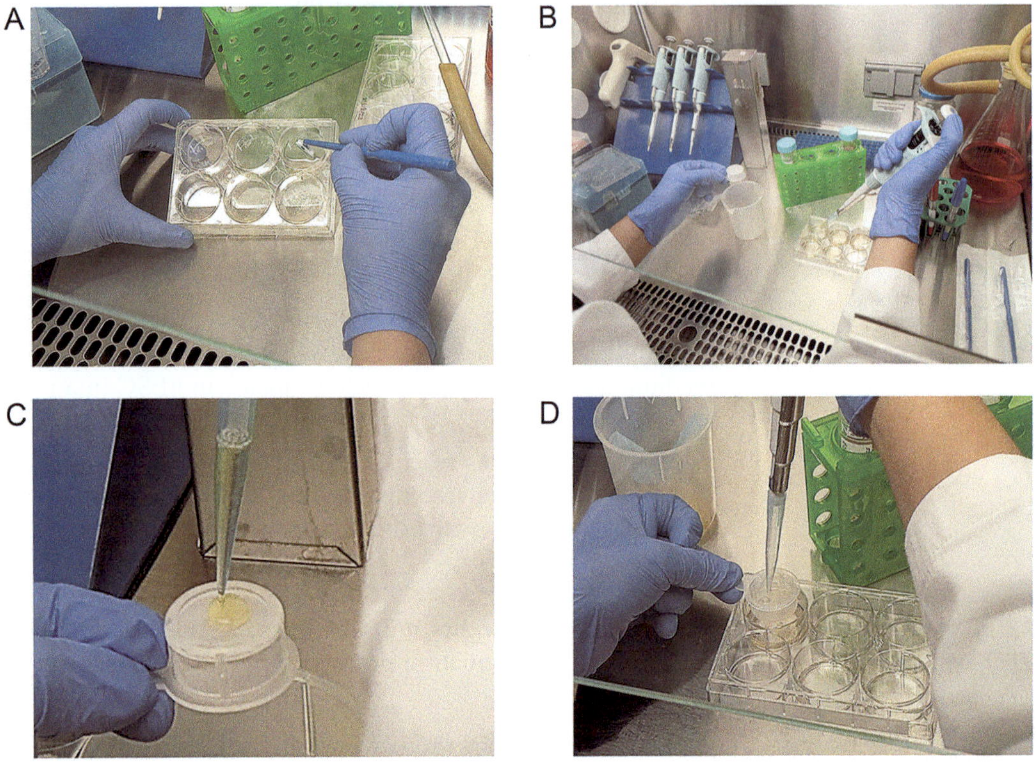

**Fig. 2** Procedure for passing hESCs and embryoid bodies onto a ultralow attachment plate. (**a**) Scrapping of hESC colonies attached onto a Geltrex-coated 6-well plate (**b**) After scrapping, hESC colonies are in suspension and can be collected with a 1000 μL pipette tip (**c**) The hESC colonies are deposited onto a 70 μm cell strainer to retain them on top of the filter (**d**) The retained colonies are gently pushed into the ultralow attachment plate using EB medium. The volumes and colonies are distributed equally along the ultralow attachment wells. This procedure is also used to change media during the EB formation

12. After 24 h (day 1), discard the EB–iROCK medium, and add 2.5 mL of EB medium (*see* **Note 6**).
13. After 48 h (day 2), replace the medium with 2.5 mL of EB medium supplemented with RA 100 nM (EB–RA medium).
14. Replace medium every 48 h with fresh EB–RA medium until day 5.
15. At day 5, replace EB–RA medium with EB medium without RA.
16. Replace medium every 48 h, until day 12, when embryoid bodies have increased in size (Fig. 3).
17. At day 12, embryoid bodies should be transferred to a Geltrex-coated 6-well plate.
18. Coat one 6-well plate with a Geltrex-DMEM/F12 solution (*see* **steps 1–4** in Subheading 3.1). From now on, these plates should no longer be of low adherence.

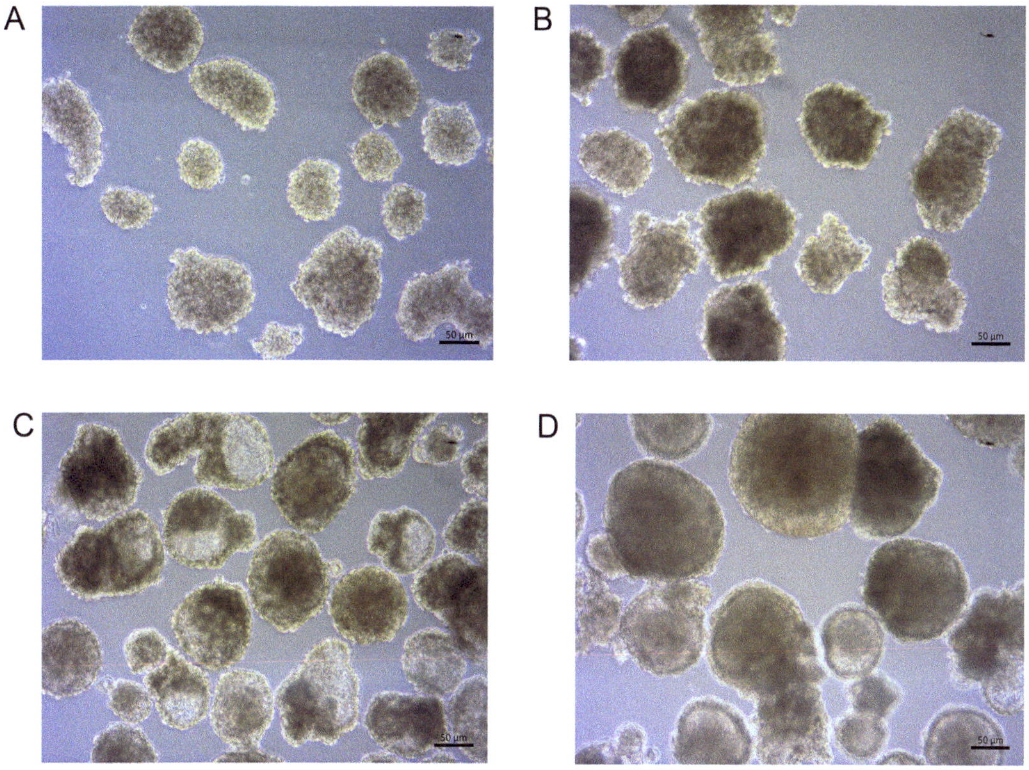


**Fig. 3** Time course of EB generation and maturation. (**a**) Early embryoid bodies 24 h after seeding in the ultralow attachment plate (**b**) EBs 4 days after seeding (**c**) EBs on day 7 after seeding (**d**) Mature embryoid bodies at culture day 11. Scale bar = 50 μm

19. For Oil Red O staining, it is recommended to seed 12-well plates, and, for RNA or protein extraction, 6-well plates are best.
20. Place the embryoid bodies in the Geltrex-coated wells using the cell strainer (Fig. 2), and add the MesenCult Adipogenic Differentiation medium to induce adipogenic differentiation.
21. Use 2 mL of MesenCult Adipogenic Differentiation medium for 6-well plates and 1 mL for 12-well plates.
22. The adipogenic differentiation medium should be replaced every 48 hours until the differentiation process is finished at day 22 (Fig. 4).

### *3.3 Lipid Droplet Staining in Adipocytes (Oil Red O Staining)*

During this procedure, sterile conditions are not necessary, although working with sterile reagents and water is recommended. This assay will stain lipids accumulated during the adipogenic differentiation.

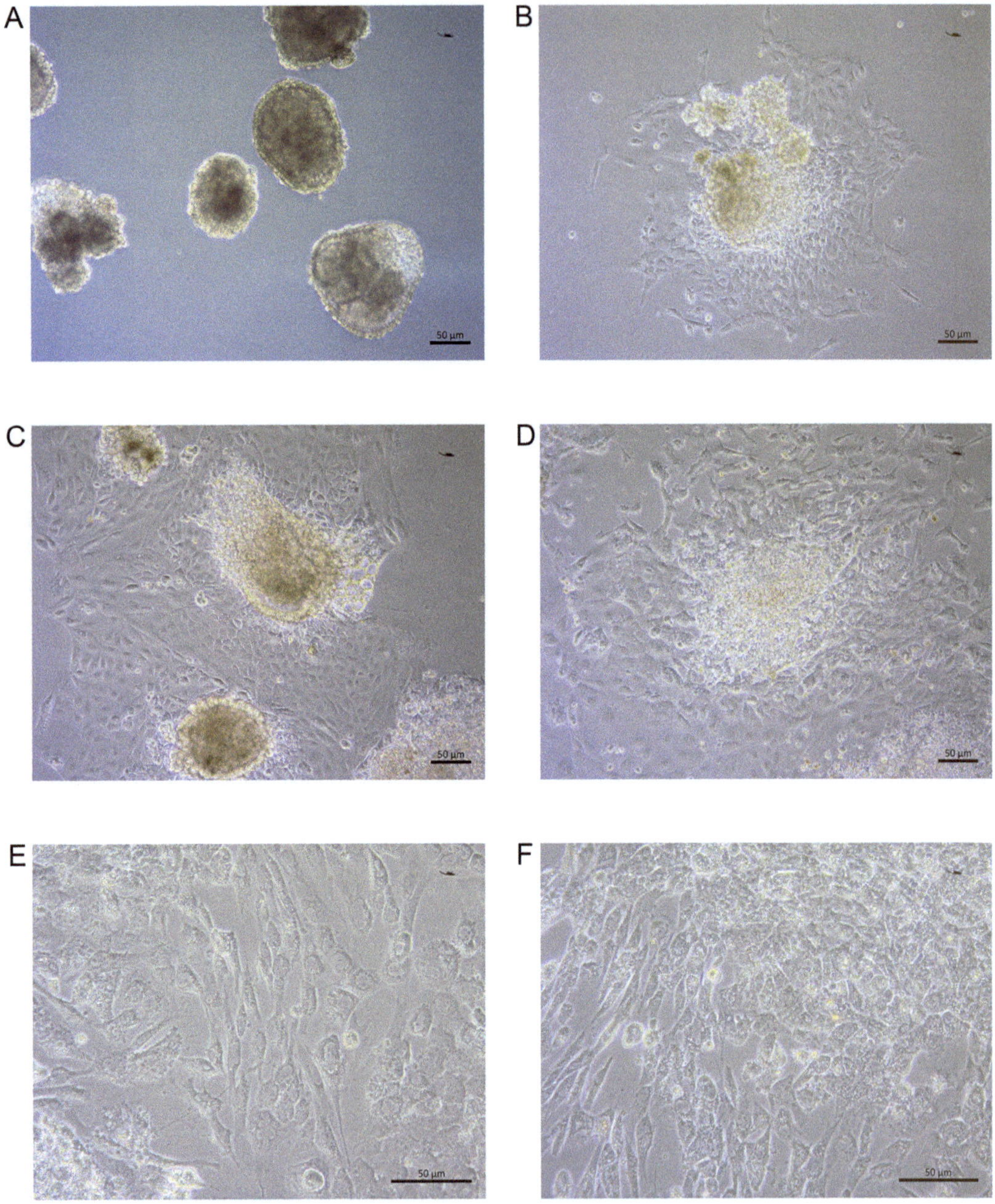


**Fig. 4** Time course of EB disaggregation and differentiation. After 12 days, EB are collected and seeded onto Geltrex-coated dishes to induce adipogenesis. This figure shows representative images of cells during adipogenesis on day 12 (**a**), day 14 (**b**), day 16 (**c**), day 18 (**d**), and at terminal differentiation on day 21 (**e**, **f**) Note that lipid droplets can be seen under the phase-contrast microscopy as bright structures inside cells

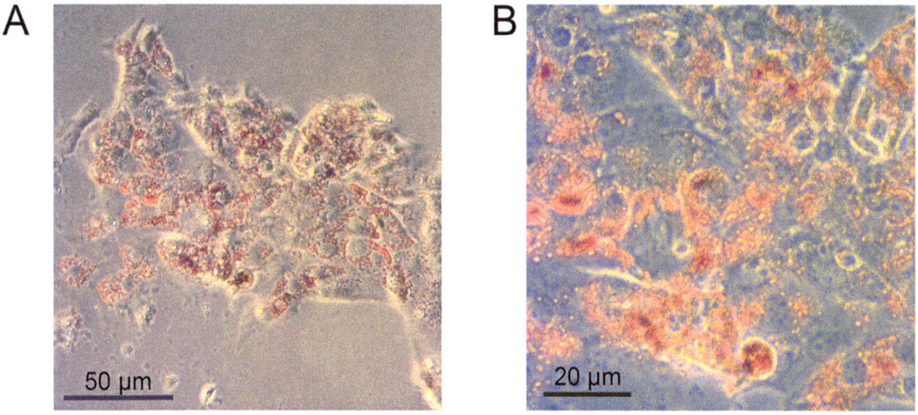


**Fig. 5** Representative images of ORO-stained adipocytes. (**a**) Magnification at 20× (**b**) Magnification at 40×

1. Remove the culture medium and wash cells twice with DPBS.
2. Carefully add 500 μL of 4% PFA solution into the walls of the well, and incubate the plate for 1 h at room temperature (*see* **Note** 7).
3. Prepare the Oil Red O solution as follows: Take 1.5 parts of the Oil Red O stock solution (*see* **step 2** in Subheading 2.3), and add one part of sterile water (e.g., mix 6 mL of the stock solution and 4 mL of water) in a 15 mL conical tube. Then, incubate the solution for 10 min at 4 °C.
4. Filter this solution through a 45 μm cell strainer, to remove precipitates.
5. Remove PFA and wash fixed cells with water (1 mL per well).
6. Add 500 μL of 60% isopropanol and incubate for 5 min at room temperature.
7. Remove the isopropanol from cells, and add 500 μL of the Oil Red O solution (prepared in **step 3**) to each well.
8. Incubate the plate for 30 min at room temperature, with gentle shaking.
9. Discard the Oil Red O solution, and rinse the cells five times with water (*see* **Note 8**).
10. Visualize and take images with a bright-field microscope (Fig. 5).

## 4 Notes

1. Geltrex is temperature sensitive, and elevated temperatures will cause the gel to rapidly polymerize and solidify. We recommend thawing Geltrex on ice and keeping it on ice during use. Upon arrival, we recommend to distribute it in 100 uL aliquots in 15 mL tubes and store it at −80 °C.

2. It is recommended to prepare a β-mercaptoethanol stock solution 100 mM, in DPBS. It can be stored at 4 °C for a month.
3. It is recommended to prepare a 100 mM RA stock solution in DMSO, which should be stored at −20 °C protected from light. Then, prepare a 1000× (100 μM) RA working solution in DPBS.
4. In case the cells do not completely detach, incubate for 1 more minute with Dispase, and wash the colonies with 1 mL of DMEM/F12. Then, add 1 mL of ESC medium, and remove carefully the colonies with a cell scraper.
5. It is essential to use the cell strainer to properly discard single cells or low-size colonies before plating in ultralow attachment plates. Embryoid bodies will not grow from single cells. To maximize collection of hESC colonies, the process of collecting and filtering hESC can be repeated with an additional 1 mL of EB–iROCK medium.
6. Since EBs do not attach to the plate, washes and medium replacement should be performed by collecting EBs with a 70 μm cell strainer, as described in **step 3** (Fig. 2b–d).
7. PFA solution should preferably be fresh or recently thawed (do not refreeze).
8. If necessary, use tap water to wash and remove precipitates or excess stain from the samples. Do not leave the samples without water; cover the samples with a lid and parafilm.

## Acknowledgment

This work was supported by the Chan Zuckerberg Initiative grant n. 2023-331942 (5022) GB-1597645 and Universidad Nacional Autónoma de México (UNAM), grant n. DGAPA-PAPIIT IN204325, to LAA. MAOS was supported by a postdoctoral fellowship from DGAPA-UNAM.

### References

1. Coelho M, Oliveira T, Fernandes R (2013) Biochemistry of adipose tissue: an endocrine organ. Arch Med Sci 9:191–200. https://doi.org/10.5114/aoms.2013.33181
2. Pant R, Firmal P, Shah VK, Alam A, Chattopadhyay S (2020) Epigenetic regulation of Adipogenesis in development of metabolic syndrome. Front Cell Dev Biol 8:619888. https://doi.org/10.3389/fcell.2020.619888
3. Sanchez-Ramirez E, Ung TPL, Alarcon Del Carmen A, del Toro-Rios X, Fajardo-Orduna GR, Noriega LG, Cortes-Morales VA, Tovar AR, Montesinos JJ, Orozco-Solis R, Stringari C, Aguilar-Arnal L (2022) Coordinated metabolic transitions and gene expression by NAD+ during adipogenesis. J Cell Biol 221. https://doi.org/10.1083/jcb.202111137
4. Zhang K, Yang X, Zhao Q, Li Z, Fu F, Zhang H, Zheng M, Zhang S (2020) Molecular mechanism of stem cell differentiation into adipocytes and adipocyte differentiation of malignant tumor. Stem Cells Int 2020:

8892300. https://doi.org/10.1155/2020/8892300
5. Yao X, Dani V, Dani C (2019) Human pluripotent stem cells: a relevant model to identify pathways governing Thermogenic adipocyte generation. Front Endocrinol (Lausanne) 10: 932. https://doi.org/10.3389/fendo.2019.00932
6. Zeevaert K, Elsafi Mabrouk MH, Wagner W, Goetzke R (2020) Cell mechanics in embryoid bodies. Cells 9. https://doi.org/10.3390/cells9102270
7. Tang QQ, Lane MD (2012) Adipogenesis: from stem cell to adipocyte. Annu Rev Biochem 81:715–736. https://doi.org/10.1146/annurev-biochem-052110-115718
8. Taura D, Noguchi M, Sone M, Hosoda K, Mori E, Okada Y, Takahashi K, Homma K, Oyamada N, Inuzuka M, Sonoyama T, Ebihara K, Tamura N, Itoh H, Suemori H, Nakatsuji N, Okano H, Yamanaka S, Nakao K (2009) Adipogenic differentiation of human induced pluripotent stem cells: comparison with that of human embryonic stem cells. FEBS Lett 583:1029–1033. https://doi.org/10.1016/j.febslet.2009.02.031
9. Zhang J, Gao Y, Yu M, Wu H, Ai Z, Wu Y, Liu H, Du J, Guo Z, Zhang Y (2015) Retinoic acid induces embryonic stem cell differentiation by altering both encoding RNA and microRNA expression. PLoS One 10: e0132566. https://doi.org/10.1371/journal.pone.0132566
10. Kam RK, Deng Y, Chen Y, Zhao H (2012) Retinoic acid synthesis and functions in early embryonic development. Cell Biosci 2:11. https://doi.org/10.1186/2045-3701-2-11
11. Kim DH, Lee J, Suh Y, Cressman M, Lee K (2020) Research note: all-trans retinoic acids induce adipogenic differentiation of chicken embryonic fibroblasts and preadipocytes. Poult Sci 99:7142–7146. https://doi.org/10.1016/j.psj.2020.09.006
12. Dani C, Smith AG, Dessolin S, Leroy P, Staccini L, Villageois P, Darimont C, Ailhaud G (1997) Differentiation of embryonic stem cells into adipocytes in vitro. J Cell Sci 110 (Pt 11):1279–1285. https://doi.org/10.1242/jcs.110.11.1279

# Chapter 2

# Quantification of Adipogenesis Using Flow Cytometry

**Carina C. Babbo, Chrisna Durandt, Melvin A. Ambele, and Michael S. Pepper**

## Abstract

Adipogenesis is a complex, multistep process by which precursor cells such as mesenchymal stromal/stem cells (MSCs) differentiate into mature adipocytes. The ability of MSCs to differentiate into adipocytes serves as a model to study human adipogenesis in vitro. Flow cytometry is a powerful technique that can be used to analyze the properties of individual cells. In this chapter, we describe a flow cytometry-based technique to quantify the proportion of MSCs that have differentiated into adipocytes.

**Key words** Flow cytometry, Adipocytes, Adipogenesis, Nile red

## 1 Introduction

Flow cytometry can be described as a technique used to analyze the physical characteristics of individual particles, mostly cells, as they flow in suspension (single file) past a light source, usually a laser [1, 2]. Cell size, cellular complexity/granularity, proteins, and intracellular organelles, which have been stained with fluorescent dyes or probes, are some of the parameters that can be analyzed using flow cytometry [2, 3]. A flow cytometer is comprised of four important components: (i) a fluidics system which aligns the cells to flow past a light source in a single file by means of hydrodynamic focusing; (ii) an optical system, which is responsible for exciting the fluorescent markers and capturing the emitted signal; (iii) an electronic component that converts the captured light signals into electronic pulses; and lastly (iv) a computer for processing and visualizing the captured data [2].

The underlying principle behind this powerful technique is the scattering of light and the detection of fluorescence emitted by individual cells. Light scatter is a nonfluorescence signal generated from laser light scattering once it hits the particle to be analyzed. Light scatter can be used to measure parameters such as cellular

Michael S. Pepper and Melvin A. Ambele (eds.), *Adipogenesis: Methods and Protocols*, Methods in Molecular Biology, vol. 2938, https://doi.org/10.1007/978-1-0716-4607-6_2,

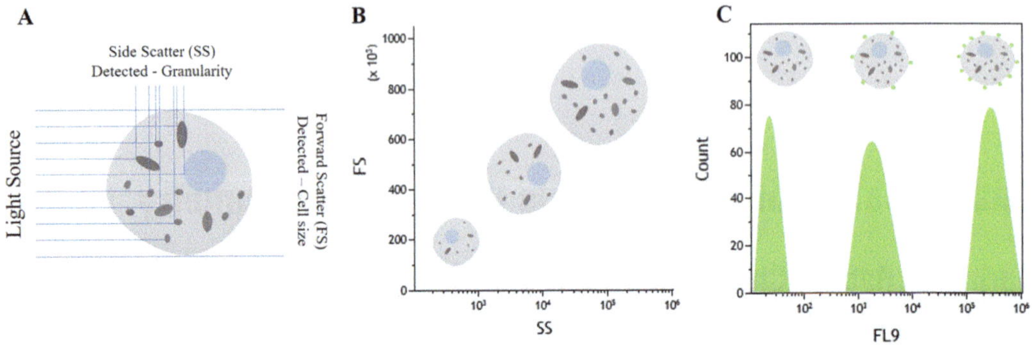


**Fig. 1** Schematic illustration of how flow cytometry makes use of scattered light and fluorescence to measure different parameters. (**a**) Schematic representation of a cell moving through a flow cytometer. Side scatter is generally a measure of cell complexity/granularity, while forward scatter is used for relative cell size determination (**b**) A plot measuring two parameters—forward scatter on y-axis and side scatter on x-axis (**c**) A plot measuring one parameter (relative fluorescence intensity). When cells are stained with a fluorescent probe such as an antibody conjugated to a fluorescent marker, the more antibodies bound to the cell, the greater the fluorescent signal emitted will be (signal shifts to the right)

complexity and cell size. There are two types of light scatter, i.e., forward and side scatter. Traditionally, forward scatter was seen as an indicator of relative cell size, while side scatter was viewed as a sensitive indicator to distinguish cells according to their morphological complexity (Fig. 1a, b). However, current views are that both side and forward scatter are indicators for cell size [4]. However, side scatter remains a more sensitive indicator of cellular complexity. On the other hand, the intensity of the fluorescence signal detected is a measure of the amount of fluorescence probe bound to a single cell [1, 2]. The signals detected are then converted to a data point, which can be visualized on a one-parameter or a two-parameter plot. A typical one-parameter plot (histogram) displays the fluorescence intensity of the signal detected on the x-axis. The counts on the y-axis represent the maximum number of events captured in the channel that accumulated the most events (Fig. 1c). The area under the histogram peak(s) represents the total number of events acquired. Two-parameter plots measure one parameter on each axis. A two-parameter plot can be divided into four quadrants, which display measurements of cell populations that are positive for both parameters, negative for both parameters, or positive for only one of the parameters (Fig. 2) [2].

An important factor to be considered when more than one parameter is being measured simultaneously, such as the detection of two cell surface markers as shown in Fig. 2, is the selection of appropriate fluorescent probes with excitation and emission wavelength that do not overlap and interfere with each other. Fluorescent compounds are excited at specific wavelengths and emit a fluorescent signal at a longer wavelength, a concept known as

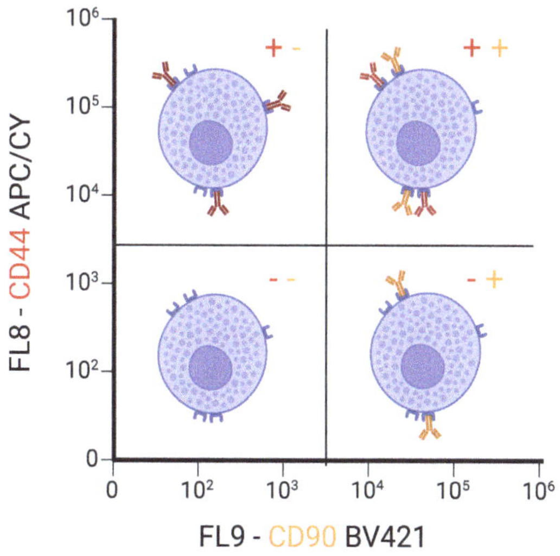


**Fig. 2** Two-parameter plot interpretation. A two-parameter plot can be divided into four quadrants, each quadrant displaying a different combination of the two parameters being measured. — = CD90−/CD44−; −+ = CD90−/CD44+; + + = CD90+/CD44+; +− = CD90+/CD44−

Stokes shift [2]. It is therefore essential to ensure that the instrument being used has a laser capable of exciting the fluorophore at the correct wavelength as well as equipped with the correct detectors to capture the emitted signal. For example, two fluorescent compounds with very similar/overlapping excitation and emission spectra cannot be placed together as it will be very difficult to distinguish between the two signals. However, when there is only a small degree of spectral overlap, compensation can be used to remove signal that has "spilled over" into unwanted channels [5]. Compensation can be defined as the process of removing interfering signal (spillover) from all detectors with exception to the detector where the signal is captured with maximum efficiency (optimal detection filter) [6].

Another essential factor to consider when performing flow cytometry is the use of controls—setup controls, specificity controls, and biological controls. Setup controls are used to ensure that the instrument is set up correctly; specificity controls are used to distinguish between nonspecific and specific binding, and biological controls are used to determine the difference between experimental conditions [7].

The following controls can be implemented:

1. Flow cytometer alignment verification fluorophores as a setup control to verify laser alignment and ensure fluidic stability.
2. Unstained cells which can be used to set up the regions in which the negative signals should appear. It is important to

note that the use of unstained cells does not control for nonspecific binding of monoclonal antibodies.

3. Isotypic controls to detect nonspecific binding/background fluorescence.
4. Untreated cells as biological controls.

One of the advantages of flow cytometry is its ability to analyze a large number of individual cells in a relatively short period of time. As cells differentiate into adipocytes, there will be an increase in intracellular lipid accumulation due to the intracellular accumulation of intracellular lipid droplets. Flow cytometry can be used to obtain a quantitative measurement of adipogenic differentiation by quantifying the percentage of cells with higher intracellular lipid levels [8]. The lipid droplets can be detected with the use of a lipophilic dye such as Nile Red, which has a high affinity for neutral lipids. However, adipocytes are fragile cells which can easily release their lipid droplets when not handled with care. Therefore, in order to exclude any free-floating lipid droplets that may have been released during sample preparation, cells can be co-stained with a nuclear stain, such as Vybrant™ DyeCycle™ (VDC) Violet (Thermo Fischer Scientific) or 4′,6-diamidino-2-phenylindole (DAPI). The advantage of using VDC Violet over DAPI is that it is membrane permeable and thus crosses the cell membrane rapidly. Using a nuclear stain in combination with Nile Red forms the basis for the flow cytometric quantification of adipogenesis protocol, as described in this chapter.

## 2 Materials

### 2.1 Reagents

1. Complete growth medium: Add 50 mL fetal bovine serum (FBS; 10%) and 10 mL penicillin (10,000 units/mL)–streptomycin (10,000 μg/mL) (Pen/Strep) to 440 mL of Dulbecco's Modified Eagle Medium (DMEM; with GlutaMAX™-I). Store it at 4 °C.
2. 0.25% trypsin-EDTA: Store it at −20 °C.
3. Nile Red (1 mg/mL): Store it at 4 °C.
4. VDC Violet (5 mM): Store it at −20 °C.
5. Absolute ethanol (EtOH), molecular grade: Store it at room temperature.
6. Flow cytometer alignment verification fluorophores: Store at 4 °C.

### 2.2 Equipment

1. Flow cytometer.
2. Centrifuge.
3. Pipette.

4. Pasteur pipette.
5. 15 mL centrifuge tubes.
6. Flow cytometry tubes.

## 3 Methods

### 3.1 Sample Preparation

1. Start with two T80 flasks and label them as follows:
   1.1 Non-induced MSCs–control cells.
   1.2 Induced MSCs/adipocytes.
2. Discard the complete growth medium in which your cells have been growing in.
3. Add 0.25% trypsin-EDTA solution to the cells, making sure it covers the entire surface of the tissue culture dish, and incubate at 37 °C for 7–10 min (*see* **Note 1**).
4. Observe cells in the flask under a microscope to make sure all the cells have detached from the bottom of the flask into a cell suspension.
5. Add an equal volume of complete growth media as the 0.25% trypsin-EDTA solution to the flask to neutralize/stop the activity of trypsin on the cells.
6. Remove 3 mL of the cell suspension using a Pasteur pipette, and transfer into a labelled 15 mL centrifuge tube.
7. Add an additional 3 mL of complete growth medium to the cells in the 15 mL tube.
8. Add 1 μL of Nile Red to 500 μL of EtOH in a 1 mL tube to make a Nile Red working solution.
9. Add 10 μL of Nile Red working solution, 1 μL of VDC Violet, and 1 mL of your cell suspension into a flow cytometry tube (*see* **Note 2**).
10. Incubate the cells for 20 min in the dark.

### 3.2 Flow Cytometry Gating and Data Acquisition

1. Switch on the flow cytometer, and acquire flow cytometer alignment verification fluorophores to verify laser alignment.
2. Acquire your non-induced cells on the flow cytometer, and follow the following gating strategy:
   2.1 Create a one-parameter plot to visualize VDC Violet positive events, i.e., nucleated cells—count vs VDC Violet/FL9 [excitation 405 nM; emission 450/40 BP]) (Fig. 3a).
   2.2 Create a two-parameter (FS Lin vs SS Log) plot, gated on VDC Violet positive events, to visualize the nucleated cells being analyzed ("Total cells" region) (Fig. 3b).

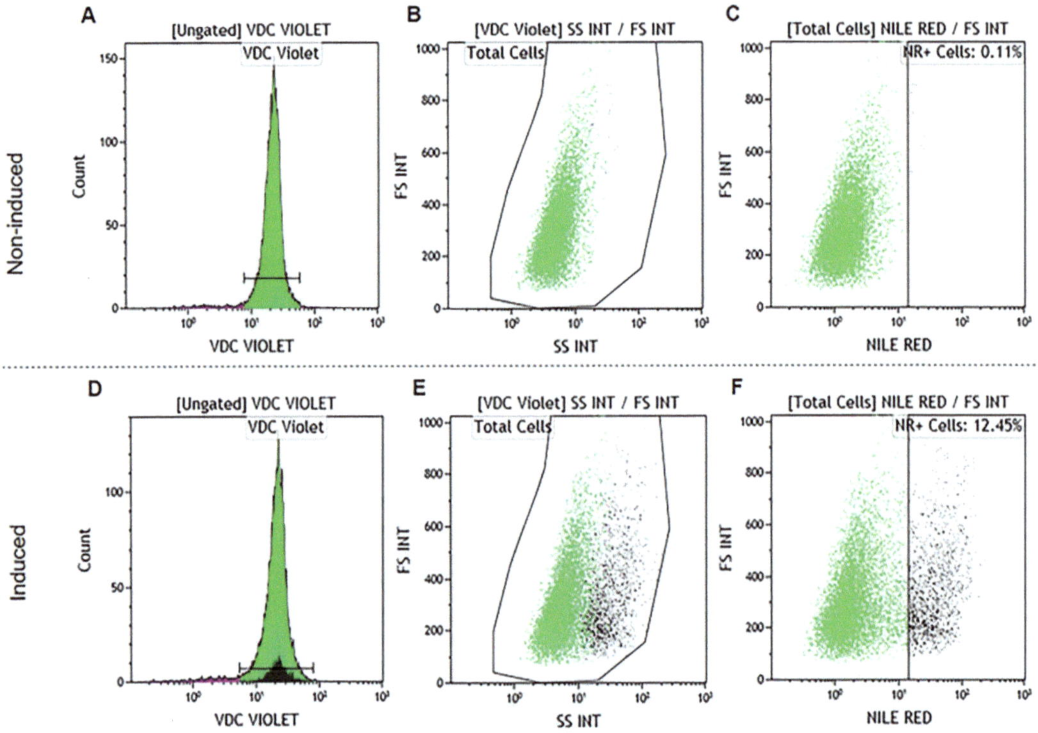


**Fig. 3** Flow cytometry set up for Nile Red assay. (**a–c**) Non-induced cells (**d–f**) Induced cells (**a, d**) VDC Violet positive events (nucleated cells) are visualized (**b, e**) Intact nucleated cells are visualized in region "Total Cells" (**c, f**) Cells which contain intracellular lipids are detected in region "NR+ Cells." The events shown in black represent cells with increased intracellular lipid levels, i.e., differentiated cells (**e, f**) The Nile Red-positive differentiated cells/adipocytes shift to the right along the y-axis of both graphs (**e**) The SS Log shift is attributed to the increasing complexity of the cells caused by the accumulation of intracellular lipid droplets

2.3 Create a two-parameter (FS Lin vs Nile Red/FL2 [excitation: 488 nM; emission 575/30 BP]) plot gated on region "Total cells" in order to determine the region in which you expect your positive events to appear ("NR+ cells" region, Fig. 3c) (*see* **Note 3**).

3. Acquire your induced cells on the flow cytometer using the abovementioned gating strategy, and collect the events in "NR + cells" region (Fig. 3d–f).

## 4 Notes

1. A total of 4 mL 0.25% trypsin-EDTA solution is enough to cover the entire surface of a T80 culture flask.

2. Use Pasteur pipettes when working with induced cells. These cells should be handled very carefully to prevent the release of the lipid droplets from the cells.
3. Save the protocol on the flow cytometer so that you do not have to set up your gates every time you run the assay.

## Acknowledgements

This research was funded by the South African Medical Research Council in terms of the SAMRC's Flagship Award Project [SAMRC-RFAUFSP-01-2013/STEM CELLS], the SAMRC Extramural Unit for Stem Cell Research and Therapy, and the Institute for Cellular and Molecular Medicine of the University of Pretoria.

### References

1. Macey MG (1988) Flow cytometry: principles and clinical applications. Med Lab Sci 45:165–173
2. Adan A, Alizada G, Kiraz Y, Baran Y, Nalbant A (2017) Flow cytometry: basic principles and applications. Crit Rev Biotechnol 37:163–176. https://doi.org/10.3109/07388551.2015.1128876
3. Wilkerson MJ (2012) Principles and applications of flow cytometry and cell sorting in companion animal medicine. Vet Clin North Am Small Anim Pract 42:53–71. https://doi.org/10.1016/j.cvsm.2011.09.012
4. Ohnuma K, Yomo T, Asashima M, Kaneko K (2006) Sorting of cells of the same size, shape, and cell cycle stage for a single cell level assay without staining. BMC Cell Biol 7:25. https://doi.org/10.1186/1471-2121-7-25
5. Szaloki G, Goda K (2015) Compensation in multicolor flow cytometry. Cytometry A 87: 982–985. https://doi.org/10.1002/cyto.a.22736
6. Roederer M (2002) Compensation in flow cytometry. Curr Protoc Cytom Chapter 1:Unit 1.14. https://doi.org/10.1002/0471142956.cy0114s22
7. Maecker HT, Trotter J (2006) Flow cytometry controls, instrument setup, and the determination of positivity. Cytometry A 69:1037–1042. https://doi.org/10.1002/cyto.a.20333
8. Durandt C, van Vollenstee FA, Dessels C, Kallmeyer K, de Villiers D, Murdoch C, Potgieter M, Pepper MS (2016) Novel flow cytometric approach for the detection of adipocyte subpopulations during adipogenesis. J Lipid Res 57:729–742. https://doi.org/10.1194/jlr.D065664

# Chapter 3

# Isolation of Wharton's Jelly-Derived Mesenchymal Stromal/Stem Cells

**Carina C. Babbo, Chrisna Durandt, Melvin A. Ambele, and Michael S. Pepper**

## Abstract

Wharton's jelly-derived mesenchymal stromal/stem cells (WJSCs) are growing in popularity as an option for cell-based therapies. These cells are found within the gelatinous matrix of the umbilical cord, referred to as Wharton's jelly. WJSCs can be isolated by enzymatic tissue digestion or by using the explant method. Here, we discuss the explant method for the isolation of WJSCs.

**Key words** Mesenchymal stromal cells, Wharton's jelly, Wharton's jelly-derived mesenchymal stroma/stem cells, Cell isolation, Cell culture

## 1 Introduction

Wharton's jelly-derived mesenchymal stromal/stem cells (WJSCs) are found within the mucoid connective tissue of the umbilical cord known as the Wharton's jelly (Fig. 1) [1, 2]. WJSCs were first isolated in 1991 by McElreavey and colleagues [3]. Since their discovery, WJSCs have gained popularity as a source of MSCs for therapeutic purposes. Several clinical trials have investigated the use of WJSCs to treat various clinical indications [2, 4].

Some advantages of using WJSCs over other stem cell sources include:

- Noninvasive harvest.
- High isolation efficiency (1–5 × $10^4$ cells/cm of umbilical cord) [5].
- There are no ethical or moral issues with sample collection.
- They are considered to be more primitive than other adult stem cells as they express a number of embryonic stem cell markers such as NANOG, DNMT3B, and GABRB3 [2, 6].

Michael S. Pepper and Melvin A. Ambele (eds.), *Adipogenesis: Methods and Protocols*, Methods in Molecular Biology, vol. 2938, https://doi.org/10.1007/978-1-0716-4607-6_3,

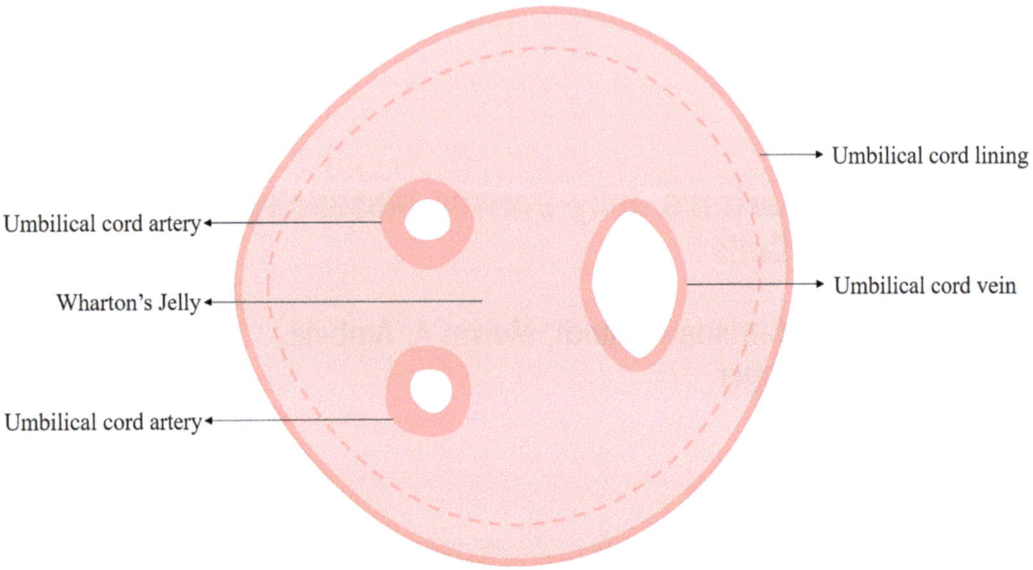


**Fig. 1** Umbilical cord cross section. The WJSCs are found within the mucoid connective tissue of the umbilical cord known as Wharton's jelly

- They conform to the ISCT guidelines for MSCs. WJSCs are positive for CD13, CD29, CD73, CD90, CD105, and HLA-ABC and negative for CD45, CD133, and HLA-DR. The positive markers occur at a frequency greater than 90%, and the negative markers occur at a frequency below 1% [6, 7].
- Non-tumorigenic and less likely to cause graft versus host disease [4].
- Can be used in an autologous or allogeneic manner [4]. WJSCs have low immunogenicity due to the low level of HLA class I and II molecules, but also due to the expression of leukocyte antigen G6 (HLA-G6), which plays a role in immune suppression [8].

## 2 Materials

### 2.1 Reagents

1. Complete growth medium: Add 50 mL of fetal bovine serum (FBS, pH 7.4) and 10 mL of penicillin (10,000 units/mL)–streptomycin (10,000 μg/mL) (Pen/Strep) to 440 mL of Dulbecco's Modified Eagle Medium (DMEM; with GlutaMAX™-I) under sterile conditions. Store the solution at 4 °C.
2. Freezing solution: Complete growth medium supplemented with 10% DMSO. For 1 mL freezing solution, add 100 μL of DMSO to 900 μL of complete growth medium.
3. Phosphate-buffered saline (PBS; pH 7.4): Store at −20 °C.

4. 0.25% trypsin-EDTA: Store at −20 °C.
5. Trypan Blue Dye: Store at 4 °C.
6. 7AAD Viability Dye: Store at 4 °C.
7. Monoclonal antibodies directed against CD34, CD36, CD44, CD45, CD46, CD90, and CD105: Store antibodies at 4 °C.
8. Dimethyl sulfoxide (DMSO): Store the solution at room temperature.

### 2.2 Equipment

1. Microscope.
2. 5% $CO_2$/37 °C water-jacked incubator.
3. Centrifuge.
4. Vacuum-assisted aspirator.
5. 15 mL tubes.
6. 50 mL tubes.
7. Tissue culture dishes (10 $cm^2$).
8. Culturing flasks (T80).
9. Flow cytometer.
10. Pipettes.
11. Scalpel.
12. Mr. Frosty™ freezing container.
13. −80 °C freezer.
14. Liquid nitrogen dewar.

## 3 Methods

### 3.1 Sample Collection

Umbilical cord samples should be collected from full-term healthy babies after obtaining informed consent.

Samples should be collected in complete growth medium to maintain viability of the cells (*see* **Note 1**).

### 3.2 Sample Preparation

1. Obtain pieces of umbilical cord that are ±10 cm in length.
2. Place the cord in a 10 $cm^2$ tissue culture dish, and rinse with pre-warmed PBS to remove as much blood contamination as possible.
3. Discard the PBS.
4. Transfer cord into a new 10 $cm^2$ tissue culture dish containing pre-warmed complete growth medium.
5. Using a sharp scalpel, cut the cord lengthwise (butterfly), and make incisions in the matrix to loosen up the tissue and expose a greater surface area of the Wharton's jelly to the surface of the culture dish.

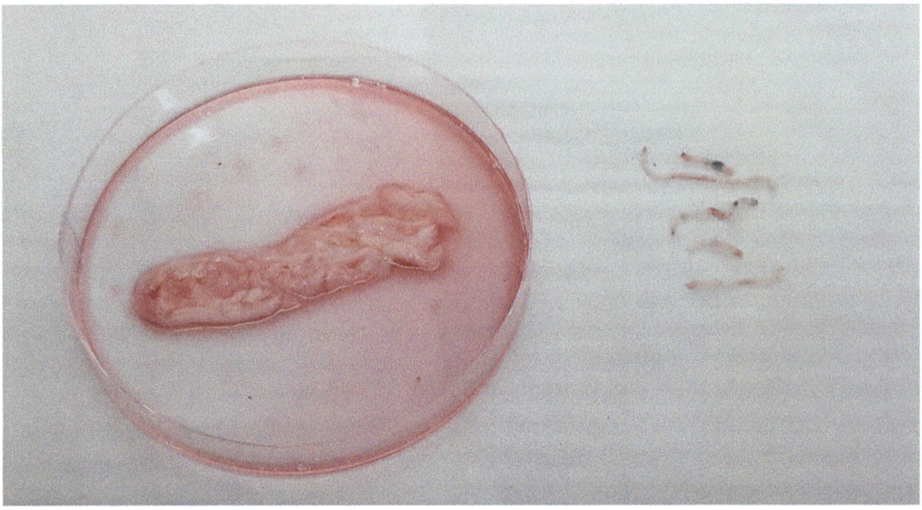

**Fig. 2** Umbilical cord sample preparation. Cut the umbilical cord lengthwise (butterfly); remove as much as possible of the blood vessels. Loosen the tissue within the umbilical cord by making small incisions in the gelatinous matrix, exposing more cells to the surface of the Petri dish

6. Carefully remove the vein and arteries to decrease the amount of blood contamination (Fig. 2).
7. Place the cord facing down in the 10 $cm^2$ tissue culture dish with pre-warmed complete growth medium.
8. Place in a 37 °C, 5% $CO_2$ water-jacked incubator. Allow approximately 3–5 days for WJSCs to migrate out of the tissue and attach to the Petri dish (*see* **Note 2**).
9. After 3–5 days, discard the umbilical cord tissue and complete culture media.
10. Add fresh pre-warmed complete growth media to the tissue culture dish, and gently swirl to help remove any remaining nonadherent cells and discard.
11. Add fresh medium and place cells back into a 37 °C, 5% $CO_2$ incubator.
12. Allow the cells to reach 80–90% confluency before passaging for further expansion or experiments.

### 3.3 Culture and Expansion of WJSCs

1. Culture the cells in a 37 °C, 5% $CO_2$ incubator until 80–90% confluence is reached.
2. Discard the complete growth medium.
3. Add 0.25% trypsin-EDTA solution to the cells, and incubate at 37 °C for 7–10 min. A total of 4 mL of 0.25% trypsin-EDTA solution should be used for T80 flasks.
4. Confirm that the cells have dislodged from the surface of the flask by observing the cells under a microscope (*see* **Note 3**).

5. Neutralize the 0.25% trypsin-EDTA solution by adding an equal volume of complete growth media to the cell suspension.
6. Transfer the cell suspension to a 15 mL or 50 mL tube.
7. Centrifuge the cells at 300 × *g* for 5 min. Discard the medium, leaving only the cell pellet in the tube.
8. Resuspend the cell pellet in complete growth media (±1 mL per T80 flask of trypsinized cells).
9. Determine the number of viable cells using the Trypan Blue exclusion assay. Take 20 μL of your cell suspension, and add 20 μL of Trypan Blue (*see* **Note 4**).
10. Add the 10 μL of stained cell suspension to the hemocytometer, and cover with the cover slip.
11. Count the number of viable cells in the four chambers. Viable cells will be the cells which did not take up the Trypan Blue dye.
12. Determine the number of viable cells per mL using the equation below:

    Equation 1: Manual cell count using Trypan Blue exclusion assay

$$\text{Cells per mL} = \frac{\text{Nr.of cells counted in the 4 chambers}}{4} \times \text{Dillution Factor} \times 10^4 \qquad (1)$$

13. Keep 300 μL of cell suspension to perform phenotype experiments.
14. Seed the remaining cells in T80 flasks at a density of $5 \times 10^3$ cells per $cm^2$, and incubate at 37 °C, 5% $CO_2$. Alternatively, freeze and store the cells if no further experiments are required.

### 3.4 Confirming MSC Phenotype and Viability Using Flow Cytometry

1. Prepare three flow cytometry tubes:
   (a) Tube 1—Unstained control.
   (b) Tube 2—Phenotype panel.
   (c) Tube 3—Viability.
2. Add 5 μL of each antibody, as listed in Table 1, to Tube 2.
3. Add 5 μL of 7AAD to Tube 3.
4. Add 100 μL of cell suspension to each flow cytometry tube (Tubes 1, 2, and 3).
5. Incubate the flow cytometry tubes in the dark at room temperature for 15 min.
6. Add 700 μL of PBS to each flow cytometry tube.

**Table 1**
**Human MSC seven-color phenotype panel example**

| Marker | Pos/Neg | Fluorochrome | Excitation (nM) | Emission (nM) |
|---|---|---|---|---|
| CD34 | +/− | Phycoerythrin/Cyanin7 (PE/Cy7) | 480, 743 | 767 |
| CD36 | + | Allophycocyanin (APC) | 650 | 660 |
| CD44 | + | Allophycocyanin/Cyanin7 (APC/Cy7) | 650, 755 | 767 |
| CD45 | − | Krome Orange (KO) | 398 | 528 |
| CD73 | + | Fluorescein isothiocyanate (FITC) | 494 | 518 |
| CD90 | + | Brilliant Violet™ 421 (BV421) | 407 | 421 |
| CD105 | + | Phycoerythrin (PE) | 480, 565 | 575 |

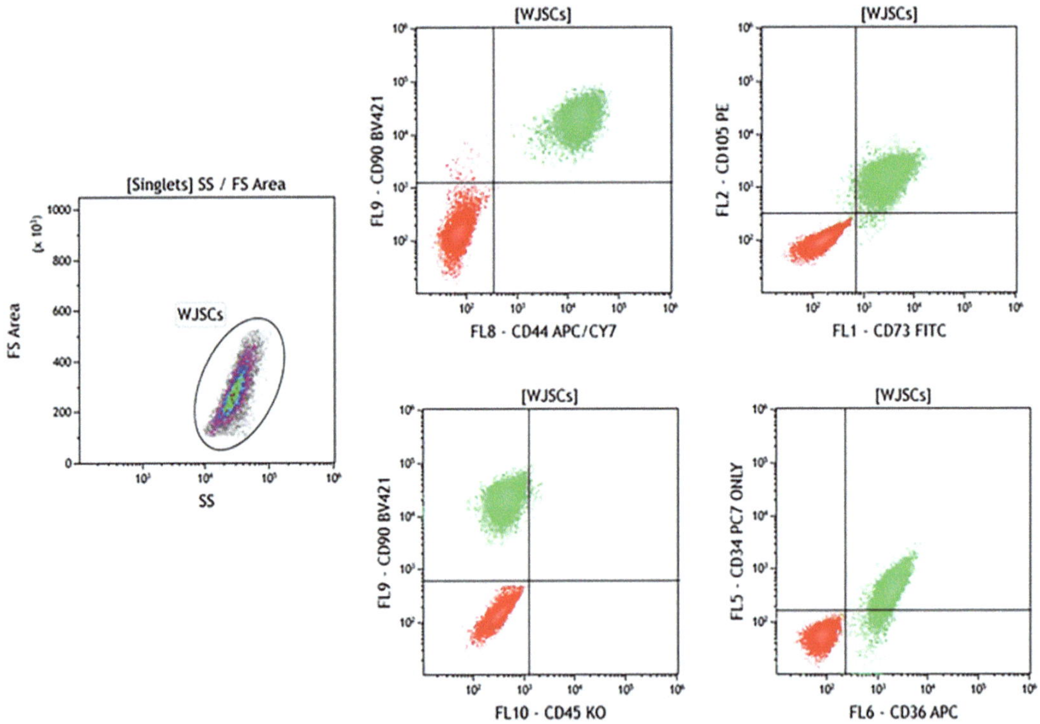


**Fig. 3** Representative overlay plots to illustrate the template used to assess the phenotypic profile of WJSCs. Input gates used are indicated at the top of each plot. Red population represent the unstained cells and were used to set the negative/positive detection boundaries. The green population represent the cells stained with the phenotype panel, i.e., representing the phenotypic profile of the WJSCs

7. Acquire all three tubes, as listed in Subheading 3.4 **step 1**, on a flow cytometer to assess the phenotype and the viability of the WJSCs. Figures 3 and 4 are representative examples of the templates used in our laboratory (*see* **Notes 5** and **6**).

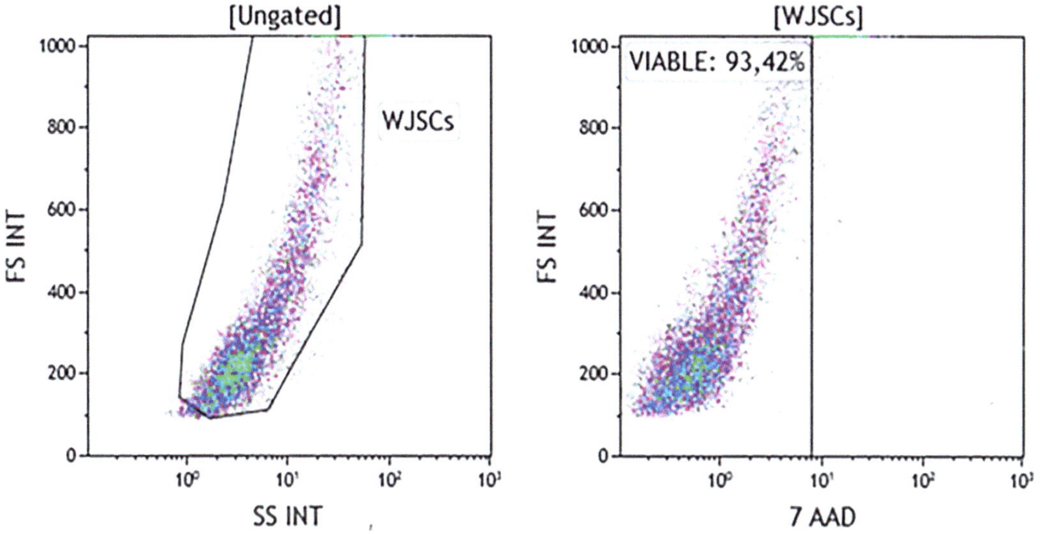


**Fig. 4** Representative density plots to illustrate the template used to assess the viability of WJSCs. Input gates used are indicated at the top of each plot

### *3.5 Freezing and Storing of WJSCs*

1. Discard the complete growth medium in which the cells have been growing.
2. Add 0.25% trypsin-EDTA solution to the cells, and incubate at 37 °C for 7–10 min. A total of 4 mL of 0.25% trypsin-EDTA solution should be used for T80 flasks.
3. Confirm that the cells have dislodged from the surface of the flask by observing the cells under a microscope.
4. Neutralize the 0.25% trypsin-EDTA solution by adding an equal volume of complete growth media to the cell suspension.
5. Transfer the cell suspension to a 15 mL or 50 mL tube.
6. Centrifuge the cells at 300 × *g* for 5 min. Discard the media, leaving only the cell pellet in the tube.
7. Resuspend the cell pellet in complete growth media (±1 mL per T80 flask of trypsinized cells).
8. A volume of 1 mL freezing solution should be prepared for every $1 \times 10^6$ cells that will be frozen.
9. Centrifuge the cells at 300 × *g* for 5 min, and discard the media, leaving only the cell pellet in the tube.
10. Resuspend the cell pellet in freezing solution ($1 \times 10^6$ cells/mL).
11. Aliquot the cell suspension into cryovials—1 mL per vial.
12. Transfer the cryovials to a Mr. Frosty™ freezing container, and store at −80 °C for a minimum of 24 h.

13. After 24 h, transfer the cryovials into a liquid nitrogen dewar for long-term storage in liquid nitrogen vapor.

## 4 Notes

1. If the collected umbilical cord is not going to be processed immediately, we recommend storing the sample in a fridge (1–5 °C) until processing.
2. During the 3–5 days that the umbilical cord is left in the incubator for the cells to migrate, check the medium daily. It may be necessary to top up the media daily to prevent nutrient depletion. Do not remove any medium; only top up to prevent the loss of any cells that have not yet adhered properly to the plastic.
3. When dislodging the cells from the flask, slight tapping on the flask may assist the cells to dislodge.
4. When determining the number of viable cells, other methods apart from Trypan Blue exclusion assay can be performed, for example, flow cytometry.
5. Instructions to generate acquisition templates are instrument (flow cytometer) specific and should be done according to the instructions-to-use guidelines provided by the supplier of the flow cytometer that will be used to do the phenotypic assessment.
6. In order to ensure accurate results, it is important to correct for any spectral spillover that may occur in a multicolor staining template. Instructions to generate a color compensation matrix, to be applied to the multicolor phenotype template, are instrument (flow cytometer) specific and should be done according to the instructions-to-use guidelines provided by the supplier of the flow cytometer that will be used to do the phenotypic assessment.

## Acknowledgements

This research was funded by the South African Medical Research Council in terms of the SAMRC's Flagship Award Project [SAMRC-RFAUFSP-01-2013/STEM CELLS], the SAMRC Extramural Unit for Stem Cell Research and Therapy, and the Institute for Cellular and Molecular Medicine of the University of Pretoria.

## References


1. Watson N, Divers R, Kedar R, Mehindru A, Mehindru A, Borlongan MC, Borlongan CV (2015) Discarded Wharton jelly of the human umbilical cord: a viable source for mesenchymal stromal cells. Cytotherapy 17:18–24. https://doi.org/10.1016/j.jcyt.2014.08.009
2. Davies JE, Walker JT, Keating A (2017) Concise review: Wharton's jelly: the rich, but enigmatic, source of mesenchymal stromal cells. Stem Cells Transl Med 6:1620–1630. https://doi.org/10.1002/sctm.16-0492
3. McElreavey KD, Irvine AI, Ennis KT, McLean WH (1991) Isolation, culture and characterisation of fibroblast-like cells derived from the Wharton's jelly portion of human umbilical cord. Biochem Soc Trans 19:29S. https://doi.org/10.1042/bst019029s
4. Abbaszadeh H, Ghorbani F, Derakhshani M, Movassaghpour AA, Yousefi M, Talebi M, Shamsasenjan K (2020) Regenerative potential of Wharton's jelly-derived mesenchymal stem cells: a new horizon of stem cell therapy. J Cell Physiol 235:9230–9240. https://doi.org/10.1002/jcp.29810
5. Kalaszczynska I, Ferdyn K (2015) Wharton's jelly derived mesenchymal stem cells: future of regenerative medicine? Recent findings and clinical significance. Biomed Res Int 2015:1–11. https://doi.org/10.1155/2015/430847
6. Nagamura-Inoue T (2014) Umbilical cord-derived mesenchymal stem cells: their advantages and potential clinical utility. World J Stem Cells 6:195. https://doi.org/10.4252/wjsc.v6.i2.195
7. Dominici M, Le Blanc K, Mueller I, Slaper-Cortenbach I, Marini F, Krause D, Deans R, Keating A, Prockop D, Horwitz E (2006) Minimal criteria for defining multipotent mesenchymal stromal cells. The International Society for Cellular Therapy position statement. Cytotherapy 8:315–317. https://doi.org/10.1080/14653240600855905
8. Vieira Paladino F, de Moraes Rodrigues J, da Silva A, Goldberg AC (2019) The immunomodulatory potential of Wharton's jelly mesenchymal stem/stromal cells. Stem Cells Int 2019:3548917. https://doi.org/10.1155/2019/3548917

# Chapter 4

# Adipogenic Differentiation Assay for the Study of Insulin Signaling

**Jonathan M. Gamwell, Emily Cresswell, and Katherine E. Pinnick**

## Abstract

In vitro models of adipogenesis are valuable tools for the study of human adipocyte development and function. Prevailing methods rely on the extended use of supraphysiological concentrations of glucose and adipogenic hormones, which can negatively impact some aspects of adipocyte function, in particular, insulin signaling. In this chapter, we present a modified adipogenic differentiation protocol which has been optimized for the study of insulin signaling and glucose uptake in human adipose-derived stem cells (hADSCs).

**Key words** Adipogenesis, Cell model, Insulin signaling, Glucose uptake

## 1 Introduction

Cell models of human adipogenesis provide accessible platforms for the study of adipocyte biology and enable cellular and molecular processes to be dissected at a resolution that may be difficult to achieve at the whole-organism level [1, 2]. Successful adipogenic cell models must have the ability to differentiate into mature, lipid-laden cells, which express the relevant adipocyte gene repertoire, and demonstrate appropriate responsiveness to physiological stimuli. As the requirements of any cell model will be unique to the specific research question, optimization of the culture conditions may be necessary to achieve translatable findings that are biologically meaningful. In this chapter, we describe an optimized adipogenic protocol that is compatible with the study of insulin signaling in human adipocytes following in vitro differentiation.

Insulin signaling in adipose tissue plays a critical role in the regulation of whole-body metabolism and energy homeostasis [3, 4]. Adipocytes are acutely sensitive to insulin, which acts to suppress lipolysis [5], while at the same time, promotes the uptake of glucose [6] and meal-derived fatty acids [7, 8], and stimulates de

Michael S. Pepper and Melvin A. Ambele (eds.), *Adipogenesis: Methods and Protocols*, Methods in Molecular Biology, vol. 2938, https://doi.org/10.1007/978-1-0716-4607-6_4,

novo lipogenesis (DNL) [3] and fatty acid esterification [9]. Perturbations in insulin signaling can contribute to a range of disease states including cardiovascular disease, type 2 diabetes, and related metabolic disorders [10]. Exploring the molecular mechanisms of insulin signaling in adipocytes not only sheds light on fundamental cellular processes but also paves the way for developing new therapeutic approaches to manage metabolic diseases.

Various techniques can be employed to evaluate the molecular and cellular responses that occur in adipocytes when insulin binds to its receptor. These include assessing the phosphorylation status of insulin signaling proteins (Western blotting, ELISA), mRNA analysis of insulin response genes, live cell imaging to visualize GLUT4 translocation, and functional assays to determine rates of glucose uptake, lipolysis, or lipogenesis. However, adipocyte cell models often display blunted insulin sensitivity and do not accurately reflect the in vivo response to insulin [11, 12]. The nonphysiological culture environment the cells are exposed to during in vitro adipogenesis can be an important determinant of this. Adipogenic culture media tend to contain supraphysiological concentrations of nutrients (e.g., glucose, glutamine) and adipogenic factors (e.g., insulin, glucocorticoids), while at the same time, they may lack some key substrates that are essential in human physiology (e.g., fatty acids).

Most protocols to induce in vitro adipogenesis require that cells are cultured in a "cocktail" of adipogenic factors for 7–14 days. Early studies, which made use of the murine 3T3-L1 cell line, were instrumental in determining the signaling pathways involved in adipocyte development and the factors required to activate them [2]. Subsequently, it has widely become the convention to include insulin, glucocorticoids (dexamethasone), and 3-isobutyl-1-methylxanthine (IBMX) in the adipogenic cocktail. PPARG agonists (rosiglitazone, troglitazone) are often added to further improve the degree of differentiation. Additional human-specific modifications include the use of serum-free media and the inclusion of other adipogenic factors like thyroid hormone (T3) [13, 14]. Across laboratories, however, the concentrations of adipogenic factors used tend not to be within physiological ranges [15], and this has the potential to alter cell behavior, limiting the translatability of findings.

In healthy human physiology, plasma insulin concentrations typically oscillate in the picomolar range (~ 20–1000 pM) [16, 17]; however, prolonged in vitro incubation with insulin (in the nanomolar range) impairs insulin signaling in various cell types including adipocytes [18–21]. Similarly, long-term dexamethasone treatment impairs glucose uptake and AKT phosphorylation in response to insulin [22, 23]. It is worth noting that chronic insulin and dexamethasone exposure are both methods used to generate models of in vitro insulin resistance [22, 24];

hence, their continuous inclusion during adipogenic differentiation may be sub-optimal for the study of insulin responses. IBMX and PPARG agonists are typically only added to the adipogenic cocktail for the first 4 days to kick-start differentiation, but there are examples of these factors being removed after 48 h rather than 96 h [25], suggesting that opportunities exist to reduce the use of adipogenic factors to improve function while still achieving successful adipogenesis.

Consideration must also be given to the nutrient composition of the adipogenic media [26]. Many basic media were originally designed with the aim of promoting cell survival rather than recreating the physiological conditions found in vivo. Glucose, for example, is often included in media formulations three to five times higher than the healthy physiological range (e.g., DMEM) [27]. There are practical reasons for this; glucose is generally the primary energy source in the culture medium, and it is essential that cells have sufficient nutrients to sustain their growth and survival. Furthermore, some cell types require a continued supply of glucose to support a higher metabolic demand. During in vitro adipogenesis, glucose can serve as a precursor for the biosynthesis of fatty acids through the process of DNL and is the primary source of glycerol for the formation of triacylglycerol [28]. However, the contribution of DNL to adipose lipid storage in vivo is relatively minor (~ 20%) [29], with the main source being the uptake of meal-derived fatty acids. Despite this, supplementation with fatty acids is not common practice in human adipogenic protocols, and this omission places artificial demands on adipocyte carbohydrate and lipid metabolism. Besides this, supraphysiological glucose concentrations can specifically impair insulin signaling in cultured cells [30, 31], yet sustained high glucose concentrations are not essential for successful adipogenesis [32].

In the following protocol, we have reduced the adipogenic media glucose concentration to 5 mM, added a physiologically relevant fatty acid mixture, and restricted exposure to all adipogenic factors (insulin, dexamethasone, IBMX, troglitazone, and T3) to the first 4 days only. hADSCs differentiated according to this protocol successfully mature into lipid-laden cells expressing adipocyte markers and are insulin-responsive [12]. We provide guidelines for assessing the insulin response in these cells by measuring early phosphorylation events in the insulin signaling cascade (insulin receptor, AKT) by Western blot.

## 2 Materials

### 2.1 Cell Culture

1. Cells: Primary or immortalized hADSCs derived from subcutaneous abdominal or gluteal adipose tissue (*see* **Note 1**).

2. Growth Medium: Dulbecco's Modified Eagle Medium/Ham's F-12 supplemented with 10% fetal bovine serum, 100 units/mL of penicillin, 100 μg/mL of streptomycin, 2 mM L-glutamine, and 0.25 ng/mL of fibroblast growth factor (*see* **Note 2**).
3. Differentiation Induction Medium (DIM): Glucose-free Dulbecco's Modified Eagle Medium/Ham's F-12 supplemented with 100 units/mL of penicillin, 100 μg/mL of streptomycin, 2 mM L-glutamine, 17 μM pantothenate, 100 nM human insulin, 10 nM triiodo-L-thyronine, 33 μM biotin, 10 μg/mL transferrin, 1 μM dexamethasone, 0.25 mM IBMX, 4 μM troglitazone, and 5 mM glucose.
4. Differentiation Maintenance Medium (DMM): Glucose-free Dulbecco's Modified Eagle Medium/Ham's F-12 supplemented with 100 units/mL of penicillin, 100 μg/mL of streptomycin, 2 mM L-glutamine, 17 μM pantothenate, 33 μM biotin, 10 μg/mL of transferrin, 5 mM glucose, and 50 μM fatty acid/BSA mixture (5 mM) (*see* **Note 3**).
5. Experimental Medium: Glucose-free Dulbecco's Modified Eagle Medium/Ham's F-12 supplemented with 100 units/mL of penicillin, 100 μg/mL of streptomycin, 2 mM L-glutamine, 17 μM pantothenate, 33 μM biotin, 10 μg/mL of transferrin, and 5 mM glucose.
6. Bovine Serum Albumin 10% Solution: Weigh out 9.5 g of bovine serum albumin (BSA; fatty acid free), and dissolve in 95 mL of glucose-free Dulbecco's Modified Eagle Medium/Ham's F-12 (*see* **Note 4**).
7. Fatty Acid/BSA Mixture (5 mM Stock): Weigh out 36.5 mg of palmitic acid powder (142 μmoles) into a glass tube. Place the tube onto a heat block, and heat at 50 °C until the palmitic acid has become liquid.
8. To the melted palmitic acid, add 121 μL (214 μmoles) of oleic acid solution (1 g in 2 mL of ethanol), 64 μL (114 μmoles) of linoleic acid solution (1 g in 2 mL of ethanol), and 5.3 μL (4.75 μmoles) of α-linolenic acid solution (250 mg in 1 mL of ethanol). Add ethanol to a final volume of 1 mL. Warm the 10% BSA solution to 37 °C.
9. In a dropwise manner, while gently swirling the 10% BSA solution in a 37 °C water bath, add the fatty acid/ethanol solution using a 1000 μL pipette (*see* **Note 5**). Leave the fatty acid/BSA mixture in a shaking water bath at 37 °C for up to 2 h to fully complex (*see* **Note 6**).
10. Use a biochemical nonesterified free fatty acids (NEFA) assay to determine the total NEFA concentration of the fatty acid/BSA mixture. Record the NEFA concentration each time a new

batch of the fatty acid/BSA mixture is prepared (*see* **Notes 7** and **8**).

11. In a biological safety cabinet, filter the fatty acid/BSA mixture through a 0.2 μm sterile filter. Aliquot into sterile tubes, and freeze at −80 °C (*see* **Note 9**).
12. Nonesterified Fatty Acids (NEFA) Assay: Use an appropriate quantitative assay for the determination of NEFA concentrations (Randox).

### 2.2 Insulin Stimulation Experiment

1. Insulin Stock Solution: Human recombinant insulin–zinc solution (688 μM) diluted to 25 μM in phosphate-buffered saline (PBS).
2. Cell Lysis Buffer: cOmplete Lysis-M EDTA-free reagent, cOmplete Protease Inhibitor Cocktail tablets, and PhosSTOP Phosphatase Inhibitor Cocktail Tablets prepared according to manufacturer's guidelines (Roche).
3. Cell scrapers.
4. Sonication probe.
5. Protein DC (detergent compatible) assay or any equivalent.

### 2.3 Sodium Dodecyl Sulfate-Polyacrylamide Gel Electrophoresis (SDS-PAGE)

1. 1× Running Buffer*:* 25 mM Tris base, 192 mM glycine, 0.1% sodium dodecyl sulfate (SDS) in 1 L deionized water, pH 8.3.
2. 10× Tris-buffered Saline (TBS): 1.5 M NaCl, 100 mM Tris base, 400 mM Tris–HCl in 1 L deionized water.
3. 1× Tris-buffered Saline with 10% Tween (TBS-T)*:* 100 mL TBS (10×), 10 mL Tween-20, 890 mL deionized water, pH 7.6.
4. 4× Loading Buffer: 10% β-mercaptoethanol in 4× Laemmli sample buffer. Aliquot and store at −20 °C.
5. TGX Stain-free Gels*:* A Mini-PROTEAN or equivalent (*see* **Note 10**).
6. Vertical Electrophoresis System: A Mini-PROTEAN Tetra Cell with a PowerPac power supply or equivalent.
7. Pre-stained Protein Ladder*:* BLUeye 10–245 kDa protein ladder.
8. ChemiDoc Imaging System.

### 2.4 Protein Transfer

1. 1× Transfer Buffer*:* 25 mM Tris base, 192 mM glycine, 10% methanol in 1 L deionized water, pH 8.3. Store at 4 °C for up to 1 week (*see* **Note 11**).
2. Transfer Membrane: 0.45 μm polyvinylidene fluoride (PVDF) membrane. Cut to size (9 × 7.5 cm for Mini-PROTEAN gels), and trim the top right-hand corner with scissors.

3. Transfer System: Criterion Blotter with buffer tank, two gel holder cassettes, four foam pads (2 per gel), a roller, and a sealed ice block.
4. Filter Paper: Thick blot absorbent filter paper, 100% cotton fiber, cut to size ($9 \times 10$ cm for Mini-PROTEAN gels), and use four pieces per gel.

### 2.5 Immunoblotting

1. Blocking Buffer: 5% skimmed milk powder in 1× TBS-T.
2. Primary Antibodies: Select primary antibodies that are reactive to the human proteins for total insulin receptor β (IR-β), total AKT, phosphorylated insulin receptor β ($pIR^{tyr1146}$) (*see* **Note 12**), phosphorylated AKT ($pAKT^{ser473}$) (*see* **Note 13**), and α-tubulin (*see* **Note 14**). Dilute each primary antibody to the recommended concentration in 20 mL of Blocking Buffer.
3. Secondary Antibodies: Horseradish peroxidase (HRP)-conjugated antibodies, raised against the host species of the corresponding primary antibody and diluted to the recommended concentration in 20 mL of Blocking Buffer.
4. Enhanced Chemiluminescent (ECL) Western Substrate: ECL substrate compatible with HRP-conjugated secondary antibodies and digital imaging.

## 3 Methods

### 3.1 Maintenance of hADSCs

For all stages of cell culture, the cells should be maintained in a humidified 37 °C incubator with 5% $CO_2$. All media and reagents should be warmed to 37 °C prior to use.

1. Maintain hADSCs in adherent cell culture flasks containing Growth Medium. Routinely passage the cells when they reach 70–80% confluency until sufficient cell number has been generated to perform the desired experiment.
2. Count the cells, and plate into 6-well adherent cell culture plates at a seeding density of $2 \times 10^5$ cells per well in 2 mL of Growth Medium. Allow two wells per sample (one labelled "basal" and one labelled "insulin treatment").
3. Incubate the cells until they are 1–2 days post-confluent (Day 0).

### 3.2 Adipogenic Differentiation

1. On Day 0, remove the Growth Media by aspiration, and replace with 2 mL of DIM.
2. On Day 2, remove the DIM by aspiration and replace with 2 mL of fresh DIM.
3. On Day 4, remove the DIM by aspiration; rinse the wells briefly with 2 mL of warm PBS, and replace with 2 mL of DMM.

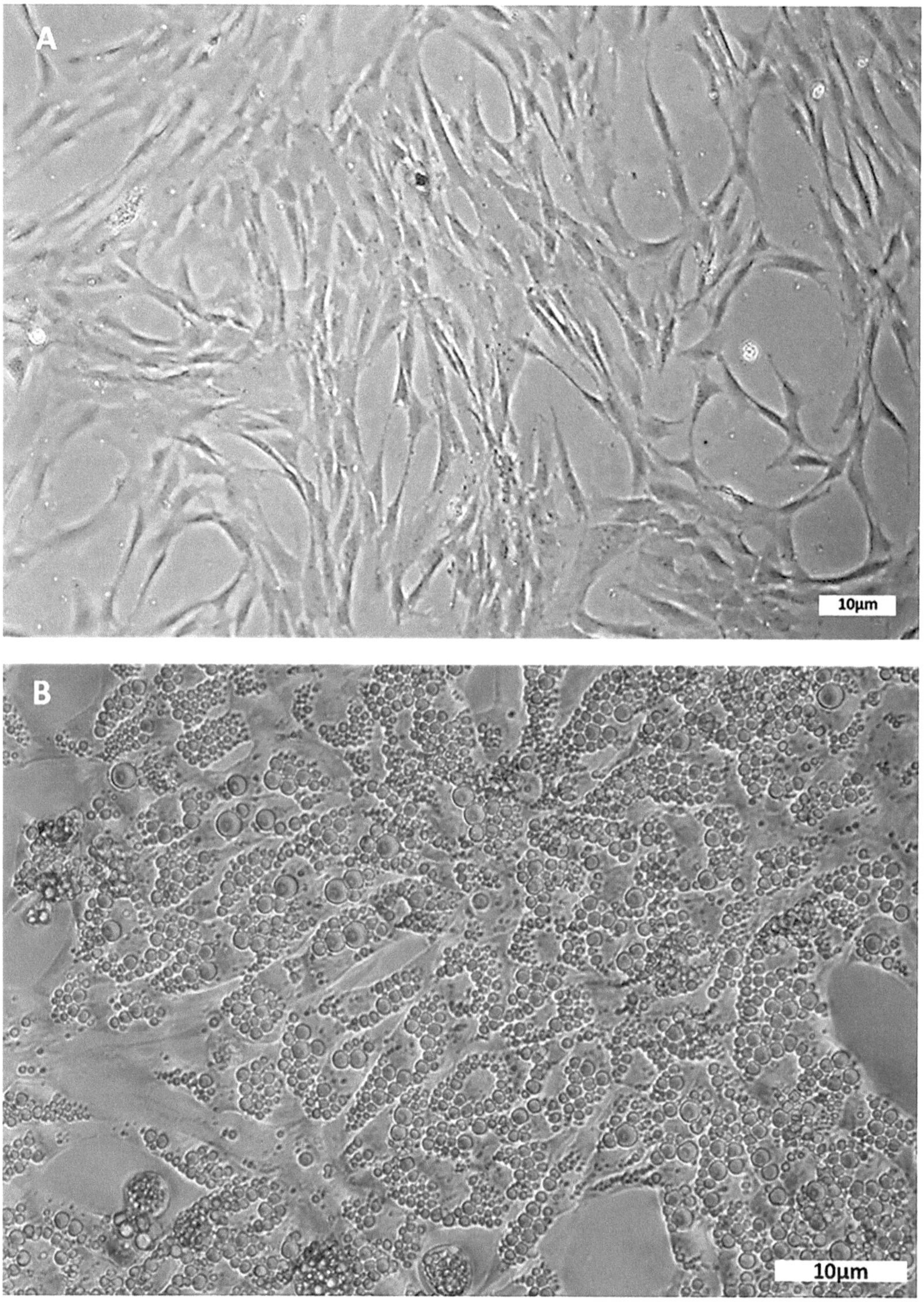


**Fig. 1** (**a**) Proliferating immortalized hADSCs in culture (magnification × 100) (**b**) Immortalized hADSCs in culture following 14 days of adipogenic differentiation (magnification × 200) (*see* **Note 15**)

4. Between Day 4 and Day 13, aspirate the DMM, and replace with 2 mL of fresh DMM every 2 days until the cells are well differentiated (*see* Fig. 1).

### 3.3 Insulin Stimulation

1. On Day 13, aspirate the DMM from all wells, and replace with 2 mL of Experimental Medium (*see* **Note 15**).
2. On Day 14 (18–20 h after the addition of Experimental Medium), add 2 μL of PBS to wells labelled "basal" and 25 nM insulin (2 μL of Insulin Stock Solution) to wells labelled "insulin treatment."
3. Return the plates to the incubator (37 °C, 5% $CO_2$) for 10 min.
4. After 10 min incubation, place the plates on ice. Remove the Experimental Medium from the wells, and rinse twice with 1 mL of ice-cold PBS.
5. Add 150 μL of ice-cold Cell Lysis Buffer to each well. Swirl to cover the cells, and incubate on ice for 5 min to lyse the cells.
6. Scrape each well using a cell scraper, and transfer the cell lysate to labelled microfuge tubes on ice (*see* **Note 16**).

### 3.4 Assess Insulin Receptor and AKT Phosphorylation by Western Blot

#### 3.4.1 Preparation of Protein Samples

1. Use a sonication probe with an amplitude setting of 34 μm to homogenize the cell lysates (*see* Subheading 3.3, **step 6**) using 3 × 5 s pulses spaced 10 s apart. After sonication, return each sample to ice immediately (*see* **Notes 17** and **18**).
2. *Optional:* Preclear the lysates by centrifuging the samples at 10,000 × $g$ at 4 °C for 10 min to pellet insoluble material. Transfer the supernatant to a new microfuge tube.
3. Determine the total protein concentration with the DC protein assay using 5 μL of samples in triplicates per sample (*see* **Note 19**).
4. Prepare 20 μg of protein aliquots in Loading Buffer for each sample (*see* **Note 20**). In fresh microfuge tubes, add the calculated volume of protein and 7 μL of 4 × Loading Buffer, and make up to a final volume of 28 μL with Cell Lysis Buffer. Briefly vortex and spin.
5. Place the tubes on a heat block and heat at 80 °C for 3 min. Allow to cool on ice.

#### 3.4.2 SDS-PAGE

1. Remove the plastic strip from the bottom of a TGX Stain-free gel, and place the gel into the electrophoresis running tank in the correct orientation.
2. Add a spacer into the opposite side of the cassette if only one gel is being run (*see* **Note 21**).
3. Add 1× Running Buffer (chilled from the fridge) to the reservoir, and check to make sure there is no leakage.

4. Briefly vortex the protein samples, and centrifuge to ensure any condensate is spun down to the bottom of the tube.
5. Load 3 μL of the Pre-stained Protein Ladder into the first and last wells and 28 μL of each protein sample into the remaining wells, taking care to avoid overspill of samples into neighboring wells.
6. After loading the protein samples, fill the main chamber of the tank to the fill line with 1× Running Buffer.
7. Replace the tank lid, and run at 100 V for approximately 2–3 h or until the dye front reaches the bottom of the gel. The protein ladder should be used as a guide to determine when the ~50 kDa marker is in the bottom portion of the gel. This ensures there will be good separation of the insulin receptor, AKT, and α-tubulin.
8. Proceed to protein transfer immediately.

#### 3.4.3 Protein Transfer

1. Remove the gel from the running tank, and carefully pry apart the panels using a cassette opening lever at the black arrow marks (*see* **Note 22**).
2. Place the gel into 1× Transfer Buffer in a shallow tray immediately.
3. Image the gel on a ChemiDoc Imaging Station using the stain-free gel settings to check that the proteins have correctly separated before proceeding.
4. Return the gel to 1× Transfer Buffer and equilibrate for 15 min.
5. Pretreat the PVDF membrane by submerging it in a shallow tray containing methanol for 1–2 min (*see* **Note 23**).
6. Pour off the methanol, and add 1× Transfer Buffer to the tray, and then allow the PVDF membrane to equilibrate in 1× Transfer Buffer for 15 min.
7. Place a transfer cassette into a shallow tray with the black side down.
8. Add a sponge pad to the transfer cassette, and fill the tray with ice-cold 1× Transfer Buffer to soak the entire system.
9. Wet two pieces of filter paper in 1× Transfer Buffer, and place them on top of the sponge.
10. Carefully transfer the gel onto the filter paper ensuring everything stays wet and that the gel is laid flat in the center. Gently roll out any bubbles with a roller.
11. Using forceps, place the methanol-treated PVDF membrane on top of the gel, keeping the trimmed corner in the top right to ensure correct orientation. Avoid moving the membrane once in contact with the gel. Roll out air bubbles gently with a roller.

12. Wet another two pieces of filter paper in 1× Transfer Buffer, and place them on top of the membrane. Add the second sponge pad (presoaked in ice-cold 1× Transfer Buffer), and roll out air bubbles with a roller.
13. Close the cassette sandwich. Submerge the entire cassette in 1× Transfer Buffer, to ensure it is entirely soaked, before placing the cassette into the transfer tank making sure to match the red side of the cassette to the red on the tank.
14. Put an ice block into the ice slot, and fill the tank with ice-cold 1× Transfer Buffer.
15. Put the lid on the tank and run at 85 V for approximately 45 min.
16. Dismantle the cassette, and, using forceps, transfer the PVDF membrane to a shallow tray containing TBS-T, and ensure the membrane is entirely submerged.
17. *Optional:* The gel and the PVDF membrane can be imaged on the ChemiDoc Imaging Station again at this point to confirm that protein transfer from the gel to the PVDF membrane has been successful and to measure total protein per sample if total protein normalization is required (*see* **Note 24**).

#### *3.4.4 Immunoblotting*

1. Transfer the PVDF membrane to a shallow tray containing Blocking Buffer (pre-warmed to room temperature), and place on a rocker for 60 min at room temperature. Ensure the Blocking Buffer covers the entire PVDF membrane for the duration of the incubation.
2. Remove the Blocking Buffer from the tray. Pick up the PVDF membrane using forceps, and use clean scissors to carefully cut horizontally across the entire membrane using the 75 kDa (red) molecular weight marker as a guide for where to make the cut. This will separate $pIR^{tyr1146}$ (95 kDa) on the upper membrane portion from $pAKT^{ser473}$ (60 kDa) and α-tubulin (50 kDa) on the lower portion. Trim the top right corner of the lower membrane portion to ensure correct orientation.
3. Place each portion of the membrane into a separate tray. Apply the $pIR^{tyr1146}$ primary antibody solution to the upper membrane portion and the $pAKT^{ser473}$ primary antibody solution to the lower portion.
4. Cover both trays with cling film and leave overnight on a rocker at 4–8 °C.
5. Transfer each membrane to a new tray containing TBS-T.
6. Place both trays on a rocker at room temperature and allow to wash for 5 min. Discard the TBS-T in each tray and replace with fresh TBS-T.

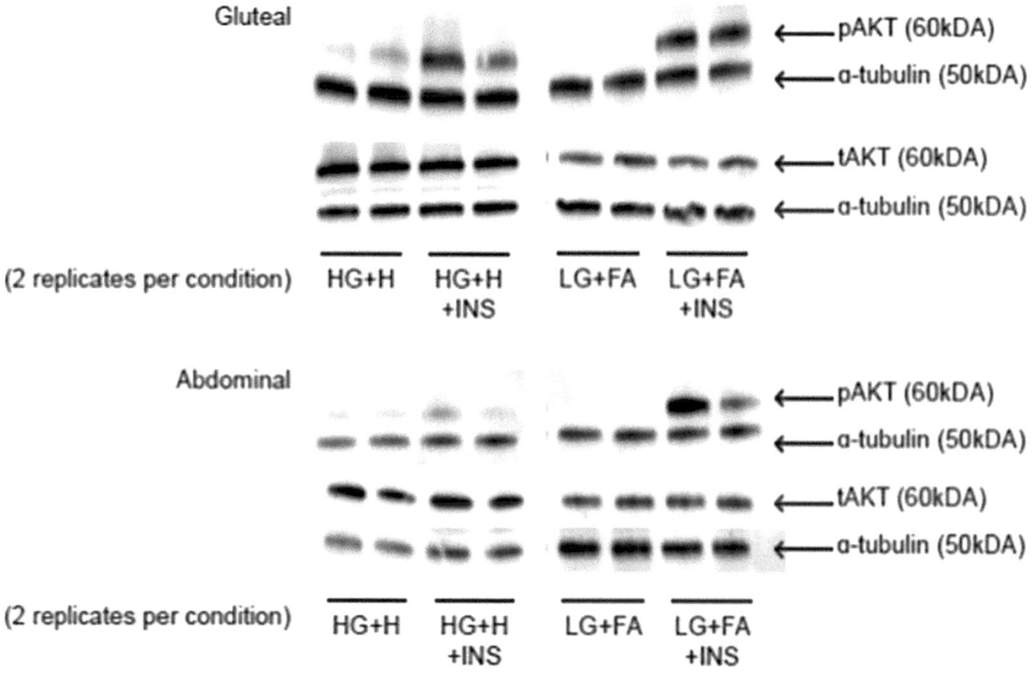


**Fig. 2** Representative Western blots showing the detection of pAKT$^{ser473}$, total AKT, and α-tubulin after 10 min incubation with either Vehicle (PBS) or 25 nM Insulin (+INS) in human immortalized hADSCs (subcutaneous abdominal and gluteal). Prior to insulin treatment, cells were differentiated for 10 days in either (**a**) high glucose (17.5 mM) and adipogenic hormone media (HG + H; containing 100 nM human insulin, 10 nM triiodo-L-thyronine, and 1 μM dexamethasone for 10 days plus 0.25 mM IBMX and 4 μM troglitazone for the first 4 days only) or according to the protocol described in this chapter in (**b**) low glucose (5 mM) and fatty acid media (LG + FA; containing: 100 nM human insulin, 10 nM triiodo-L-thyronine, 1 μM dexamethasone, 0.25 mM IBMX, and 4 μM troglitazone for the first 4 days only). (Figure adapted from [12] (CC BY 4.0))

7. Repeat **step 6** three more times.
8. Transfer each membrane to a new tray, and add the corresponding Secondary Antibody solutions. Place both trays on a rocker at room temperature for 60 min.
9. Remove and discard the Secondary Antibody solutions. Transfer each membrane to a new tray containing TBS-T.
10. Place both trays on a rocker at room temperature and allow to wash for 5 min. Discard the TBS-T in each tray and replace with fresh TBS-T.
11. Repeat **step 10** three times.
12. Prepare 3 mL ECL substrate per membrane, working in the dark. Do so by mixing equal parts of the peroxide solution and Luminol/Enhancer reagent shortly before use to ensure equilibration and protect the ECL substrate from the light.
13. For the pIR$^{tyr1146}$ portion of the membrane, pour off the last TBS-T wash (**step 11**), and blot the membrane gently against

the side of the tray to remove any remaining TBS-T before transferring to a new tray.

14. Cover the membrane evenly with ECL substrate, and incubate for 2–3 min, at room temperature and in the dark. Halfway through the incubation period, turn the membrane over and gently agitate the tray. Turn the membrane over in this way three to four times until the end of the incubation.
15. Using forceps, gently shake off the excess ECL substrate, and transfer the membrane to a clean tray.
16. Transport the membrane to the ChemiDoc Imaging Station, and image using the Chemi Blot settings.
17. Repeat **steps 13–16** for the $pAKT^{ser473}/\alpha$-tubulin portion of the membrane (*see* Fig. 2).
18. After imaging $pAKT^{ser473}$, transfer the membrane to a clean tray containing TBS-T, and place the tray on a rocker at room temperature, and allow to wash for 5 min.
19. Discard the TBS-T and replace with fresh TBS-T. Repeat this step three more times.
20. Repeat **steps 8–16** using the α-tubulin Primary Antibody solution and corresponding Secondary Antibody.

## 4 Notes

1. Further optimization not indicated here may be required for cells derived from other adipose depots (e.g., visceral) or sources (e.g., other species or cell lines).
2. Dulbecco's Modified Eagle Medium/Ham's F-12 contains 17.5 mM glucose in the formulation.
3. In humans, the typical daily range for plasma NEFA is 100–700 μM [33]. The final concentration of fatty acids added to the DMM is at the lower end of this range. This is to avoid difficulties with cell floating/lifting, which can become an issue if the cells become overladen with lipid and buoyant.
4. Prepare the 10% BSA solution in a glass bottle, and warm the solution to 37 °C before use.
5. It is important to work continuously and to ensure the drops are uniform in size. If the drops are too large, fatty acids may precipitate when entering the BSA solution. If there is any sign of wax forming in the pipette tip, return the tube and pipette tip briefly to the heat block until the wax has melted.
6. The final ratio of fatty acids complexed to BSA is 3:1. In healthy humans, the ratio of serum fatty acids to albumin ranges from 1:1 to 3:1 [34].

7. If the measured NEFA concentration is more than 10% outside the target, then the fatty acid/BSA mixture should be remade to ensure the correct 3:1 ratio of fatty acids to BSA.
8. The proportion of each fatty acid species in the fatty acid/BSA mixture is as follows: oleic acid (45%), palmitic acid (30%), linoleic acid (24%), and α-linolenic acid (1%). This is representative of the proportions of the most abundant fatty acids found in healthy human serum [35]. α-Linolenic acid is included because it is an essential fatty acid, meaning that it cannot be synthesized by human cells, and must therefore be supplemented to culture media.
9. Avoid multiple freeze–thaw cycles of the fatty acid/BSA mixture. The fatty acid composition of plasma lipids has been shown to be stable for up to 4 years when stored at −80 °C [36].
10. An acrylamide percentage of 7.5% is recommended to give reasonable separation between bands for the insulin receptor (95 kDa), AKT (60 kDa), and α-tubulin (50 kDa).
11. The 1× Transfer Buffer should be stored at 4–8 °C so that it is cold when added to the transfer tank. This is because heat will be generated during the transfer process.
12. Autophosphorylation of tyrosine residues in the insulin receptor β-subunits is one of the earliest events in the molecular response to insulin and begins with phosphorylation of tyrosine residue 1146 (Tyr1146) [37]. Insulin receptors share significant structural and functional homology with IGF-1 receptors, so some antibodies may also detect phosphorylation of Tyr1131 of the IGF-1 receptor [38].
13. AKT is an insulin-signaling protein downstream of the insulin receptor that is activated by phosphorylation of serine residue 473 (ser473) within the carboxy terminus [39].
14. α-Tubulin serves as the internal loading control. The target proteins are expressed relative to α-tubulin to overcome small differences in sample loading and lane variation. It is assumed that the amount of α-tubulin detected will be directly proportional to the total amount of protein in the sample. Preliminary experiments should be performed to confirm the internal loading control is stably expressed across all the experimental conditions as the expression may be affected by cell type or treatment.
15. It is advisable to inspect cell cultures at Day 13 prior to commencing insulin stimulation. Successful adipogenic differentiation is confirmed by the change in morphology from thin, fibroblast-like cells to enlarged cells filled with lipid droplets. If required, additional cell samples can be harvested at this

point to measure intracellular triacylglycerol and adipogenic gene expression, as previously described [12].

16. Cell lysates can be stored at −80 °C. If protein samples have been stored at −80 °C, thaw the tubes on ice. Once completely thawed, vortex samples, and briefly spin in a microcentrifuge to ensure all condensate is spun down. Place tubes back on ice.
17. At this step, it is important to avoid overprocessing and sample foaming or splashing. Ensure the sonicator probe tip is submerged at least 0.5 cm below the surface of liquid and does not touch the bottom or sides of the tube.
18. Sonication generates heat which can denature proteins. To avoid this, ensure the sample is kept on ice between pulses when sonicating.
19. Prepare the protein standard curve using the Cell Lysis Buffer as the diluent.
20. It is advisable that multiple protein samples are aliquoted and stored in Loading Buffer at −80 °C from this point to avoid repeated freeze–thawing of the entire sample, which can lead to protein degradation.
21. $pIR^{tyr1146}$ and $pAKT^{ser473}$ must be run on a separate gel to total IR-β and total AKT. If desired, both gels can be run together in parallel at this point. Alternatively, the SDS-PAGE, protein transfer, and immunoblotting steps must be repeated separately for total IR-β and total AKT.
22. It can be useful at this point to trim a corner of the gel using a metal spatula to ensure correct orientation of the gel lanes.
23. When handling the PVDF membrane, always use forceps, and avoid touching with gloves.
24. The use of stain-free blot settings allows total protein to be measured on the PVDF membrane for each sample. Total protein normalization is increasingly becoming the gold standard as it eliminates the need for internal loading controls, which may not be stably expressed, and it accounts for variation in transfer efficiency. Normalization settings are available within the ChemiDoc software to calculate band intensity relative to total protein lane intensity.

## References

1. Ruiz-Ojeda FJ, Ruperez AI, Gomez-Llorente-C, Gil A, Aguilera CM (2016) Cell models and their application for studying Adipogenic differentiation in relation to obesity: a review. Int J Mol Sci 17:ARTN 1040. https://doi.org/10.3390/ijms17071040
2. Dufau J, Shen JX, Couchet M, Barbosa TD, Mejhert N, Massier L, Griseti E, Mouisel E, Amri EZ, Lauschke VM, Ryden M, Langin D (2021) In vitro and ex vivo models of adipocytes. Am J Phys Cell Phys 320:C822–C841. https://doi.org/10.1152/ajpcell.00519.2020

3. Santoro A, McGraw TE, Kahn BB (2021) Insulin action in adipocytes, adipose remodeling, and systemic effects. Cell Metab 33:748–757. https://doi.org/10.1016/j.cmet.2021.03.019
4. Petersen MC, Shulman GI (2018) Mechanisms of insulin action and insulin resistance. Physiol Rev 98:2133–2223. https://doi.org/10.1152/physrev.00063.2017
5. Bolinder J, Kager L, Ostman J, Arner P (1983) Differences at the receptor and postreceptor levels between human omental and subcutaneous adipose tissue in the action of insulin on lipolysis. Diabetes 32:117–123. https://doi.org/10.2337/diab.32.2.117
6. Hagstrom-Toft E, Arner P, Johansson U, Eriksson LS, Ungerstedt U, Bolinder J (1992) Effect of insulin on human adipose tissue metabolism in situ. Interactions with beta-adrenoceptors. Diabetologia 35:664–670. https://doi.org/10.1007/BF00400260
7. Yki-Jarvinen H, Taskinen MR, Koivisto VA, Nikkila EA (1984) Response of adipose tissue lipoprotein lipase activity and serum lipoproteins to acute hyperinsulinaemia in man. Diabetologia 27:364–369. https://doi.org/10.1007/BF00304851
8. Stahl A, Evans JG, Pattel S, Hirsch D, Lodish HF (2002) Insulin causes fatty acid transport protein translocation and enhanced fatty acid uptake in adipocytes. Dev Cell 2:477–488. https://doi.org/10.1016/s1534-5807(02)00143-0
9. Czech MP, Tencerova M, Pedersen DJ, Aouadi M (2013) Insulin signalling mechanisms for triacylglycerol storage. Diabetologia 56:949–964. https://doi.org/10.1007/s00125-013-2869-1
10. White MF, Kahn CR (2021) Insulin action at a molecular level – 100 years of progress. Mol Metab 52:101304. https://doi.org/10.1016/j.molmet.2021.101304
11. Friesen M, Khalil AS, Barrasa MI, Jeppesen JF, Mooney DJ, Jaenisch R (2022) Development of a physiological insulin resistance model in human stem cell-derived adipocytes. Sci Adv 8:eabn7298. https://doi.org/10.1126/sciadv.abn7298
12. Gamwell JM, Paphiti K, Hodson L, Karpe F, Pinnick KE, Todorcevic M (2023) An optimised protocol for the investigation of insulin signalling in a human cell culture model of adipogenesis. Adipocytes 12:2179339. https://doi.org/10.1080/21623945.2023.2179339
13. Hauner H, Skurk T, Wabitsch M (2001) Cultures of human adipose precursor cells. Methods Mol Biol 155:239–247. https://doi.org/10.1385/1-59259-231-7:239
14. Lee MJ, Fried SK (2014) Optimal protocol for the differentiation and metabolic analysis of human adipose stromal cells. Methods Enzymol 538:49–65. https://doi.org/10.1016/B978-0-12-800280-3.00004-9
15. Scott MA, Nguyen VT, Levi B, James AW (2011) Current methods of adipogenic differentiation of mesenchymal stem cells. Stem Cells Dev 20:1793–1804. https://doi.org/10.1089/scd.2011.0040
16. Polonsky KS, Given BD, Van Cauter E (1988) Twenty-four-hour profiles and pulsatile patterns of insulin secretion in normal and obese subjects. J Clin Invest 81:442–448. https://doi.org/10.1172/JCI113339
17. Pramfalk C, Pavlides M, Banerjee R, McNeil CA, Neubauer S, Karpe F, Hodson L (2016) Fasting plasma insulin concentrations are associated with changes in hepatic fatty acid synthesis and partitioning prior to changes in liver fat content in healthy adults. Diabetes 65:1858–1867. https://doi.org/10.2337/db16-0236
18. Nelson BA, Robinson KA, Buse MG (2002) Defective Akt activation is associated with glucose- but not glucosamine-induced insulin resistance. Am J Physiol Endocrinol Metab 282:E497–E506. https://doi.org/10.1152/ajpendo.00438.2001
19. Rossi A, Eid M, Dodgson J, Davies G, Musial B, Wabitsch M, Church C, Hornigold DC (2020) In vitro characterization of the effects of chronic insulin stimulation in mouse 3T3-L1 and human SGBS adipocytes. Adipocytes 9:415–426. https://doi.org/10.1080/21623945.2020.1798613
20. De Nigris V, Pujadas G, La Sala L, Testa R, Genovese S, Ceriello A (2015) Short-term high glucose exposure impairs insulin signaling in endothelial cells. Cardiovasc Diabetol 14: ARTN 114. https://doi.org/10.1186/s12933-015-0278-0
21. Bertacca A, Ciccarone A, Cecchetti P, Vianello B, Laurenza I, Maffei M, Chiellini C, Del Prato S, Benzi L (2005) Continually high insulin levels impair Akt phosphorylation and glucose transport in human myoblasts. Metabolism 54:1687–1693. https://doi.org/10.1016/j.metabol.2005.06.019
22. Lo KA, Labadorf A, Kennedy NJ, Han MS, Yap YS, Matthews B, Xin X, Sun L, Davis RJ, Lodish HF, Fraenkel E (2013) Analysis of in vitro insulin-resistance models and their physiological relevance to in vivo diet-induced adipose insulin resistance. Cell Rep 5:259–270. https://doi.org/10.1016/j.celrep.2013.08.039

23. Tan SX, Fisher-Wellman KH, Fazakerley DJ, Ng Y, Pant H, Li J, Meoli CC, Coster AC, Stockli J, James DE (2015) Selective insulin resistance in adipocytes. J Biol Chem 290: 11337–11348. https://doi.org/10.1074/jbc.M114.623686
24. Yudhani RD, Sari Y, Nugrahaningsih DAA, Sholikhah EN, Rochmanti M, Purba AKR, Khotimah H, Nugrahenny D, Mustofa M (2023) In vitro insulin resistance model: a recent update. J Obes 2023:1964732. https://doi.org/10.1155/2023/1964732
25. Park BO, Ahrends R, Teruel MN (2012) Consecutive positive feedback loops create a bistable switch that controls preadipocyte-to-adipocyte conversion. Cell Rep 2:976–990. https://doi.org/10.1016/j.celrep.2012.08.038
26. Lagziel S, Gottlieb E, Shlomi T (2020) Mind your media. Nat Metab 2:1369–1372. https://doi.org/10.1038/s42255-020-00299-y
27. McKee TJ, Komarova SV (2017) Is it time to reinvent basic cell culture medium? Am J Physiol Cell Physiol 312:C624–C626. https://doi.org/10.1152/ajpcell.00336.2016
28. Collins JM, Neville MJ, Pinnick KE, Hodson L, Ruyter B, van Dijk TH, Reijngoud DJ, Fielding MD, Frayn KN (2011) De novo lipogenesis in the differentiating human adipocyte can provide all fatty acids necessary for maturation. J Lipid Res 52:1683–1692. https://doi.org/10.1194/jlr.M012195
29. Strawford A, Antelo F, Christiansen M, Hellerstein MK (2004) Adipose tissue triglyceride turnover, de novo lipogenesis, and cell proliferation in humans measured with (H2O)-H-2. Am J Physiol Endocrinol Metab 286:E577–E588. https://doi.org/10.1152/ajpendo.00093.2003
30. Palacios-Ortega S, Varela-Guruceaga M, Martinez JA, de Miguel C, Milagro FI (2016) Effects of high glucose on caveolin-1 and insulin signaling in 3T3-L1 adipocytes. Adipocytes 5:65–80. https://doi.org/10.1080/21623945.2015.1122856
31. Oku A, Nawano M, Ueta K, Fujita T, Umebayashi I, Arakawa K, Kano-Ishihara T, Saito A, Anai M, Funaki M, Kikuchi M, Oka Y, Asano T (2001) Inhibitory effect of hyperglycemia on insulin-induced Akt/protein kinase B activation in skeletal muscle. Am J Physiol Endocrinol Metab 280:E816–E824. https://doi.org/10.1152/ajpendo.2001.280.5.E816
32. Jackson RM, Griesel BA, Gurley JM, Szweda LI, Olson AL (2017) Glucose availability controls adipogenesis in mouse 3T3-L1 adipocytes via up-regulation of nicotinamide metabolism. J Biol Chem 292:18556–18564. https://doi.org/10.1074/jbc.M117.791970
33. Frayn KN, Williams CM, Arner P (1996) Are increased plasma non-esterified fatty acid concentrations a risk marker for coronary heart disease and other chronic diseases? Clin Sci (Lond) 90:243–253. https://doi.org/10.1042/cs0900243
34. Alsabeeh N, Chausse B, Kakimoto PA, Kowaltowski AJ, Shirihai O (2018) Cell culture models of fatty acid overload: problems and solutions. Biochim Biophys Acta Mol Cell Biol Lipids 1863:143–151. https://doi.org/10.1016/j.bbalip.2017.11.006
35. Hodson L, Skeaff CM, Fielding BA (2008) Fatty acid composition of adipose tissue and blood in humans and its use as a biomarker of dietary intake. Prog Lipid Res 47:348–380. https://doi.org/10.1016/j.plipres.2008.03.003
36. Hodson L, Skeaff CM, Wallace AJ, Arribas GL (2002) Stability of plasma and erythrocyte fatty acid composition during cold storage. Clin Chim Acta 321:63–67. https://doi.org/10.1016/s0009-8981(02)00100-6
37. White MF, Shoelson SE, Keutmann H, Kahn CR (1988) A cascade of tyrosine autophosphorylation in the beta-subunit activates the phosphotransferase of the insulin receptor. J Biol Chem 263:2969–2980. https://doi.org/10.1016/S0021-9258(18)69163-X
38. Abbott AM, Bueno R, Pedrini MT, Murray JM, Smith RJ (1992) Insulin-like growth factor I receptor gene structure. J Biol Chem 267: 10759–10763. https://doi.org/10.1016/S0021-9258(19)50083-7
39. Alessi DR, Andjelkovic M, Caudwell B, Cron P, Morrice N, Cohen P, Hemmings BA (1996) Mechanism of activation of protein kinase B by insulin and IGF-1. EMBO J 15:6541–6551

# Chapter 5

## Quantification of Lipid Droplets in Adipocytes

**Reabetswe R. Pitere, Carina C. Babbo, Rachel Giles, Melvin A. Ambele, and Michael S. Pepper**

### Abstract

Lipid droplets are cellular organelles that regulate various cellular process such as lipid and energy metabolism. The first morphological indication of adipogenesis is the accumulation of multiple small intracellular lipid droplets. Here, we describe a microscopy technique that can be used to quantify lipid droplets in adipocytes.

**Key words** ASCs, Adipocyte, Adipogenesis, Adipogenic differentiation, Lipid quantification

## 1 Introduction

Lipid droplets are intracellular and multifunctional organelles in the cytosol that are important for storing lipids and maintaining energy homeostasis [1]. In addition, they are crucial for regulating thermogenic activity and cellular metabolism, alleviating cellular stress, and facilitating communication between different organelles [1–3]. Lipid droplets are composed of a core of neutral lipids (consisting mainly of triacylglycerols and sterol esters), which are enclosed by a monolayer of phospholipids and other proteins [4]. Lipid droplets are abundant in adipose tissue cells. They are synthesized by the endoplasmic reticulum and interact with other cellular organelles through membrane contact sites [4, 5]. During adipogenesis in vitro, the mature adipocyte differentiated from adipose-derived stem/stromal cells (ASCs) is characterized by the formation of lipid droplets [6]. Small intracellular lipid droplets will form, which will eventually merge into one unilocular lipid droplet as the preadipocyte cells mature into adipocytes (Fig. 1).

Intracellular accumulation of lipid droplets is associated with a range of diseases including obesity, hepatic steatosis, coronary artery diseases, and cancer [1, 7]. Quantification of lipid droplets is important in understanding changes in lipid metabolism, and

Michael S. Pepper and Melvin A. Ambele (eds.), *Adipogenesis: Methods and Protocols*, Methods in Molecular Biology, vol. 2938, https://doi.org/10.1007/978-1-0716-4607-6_5,

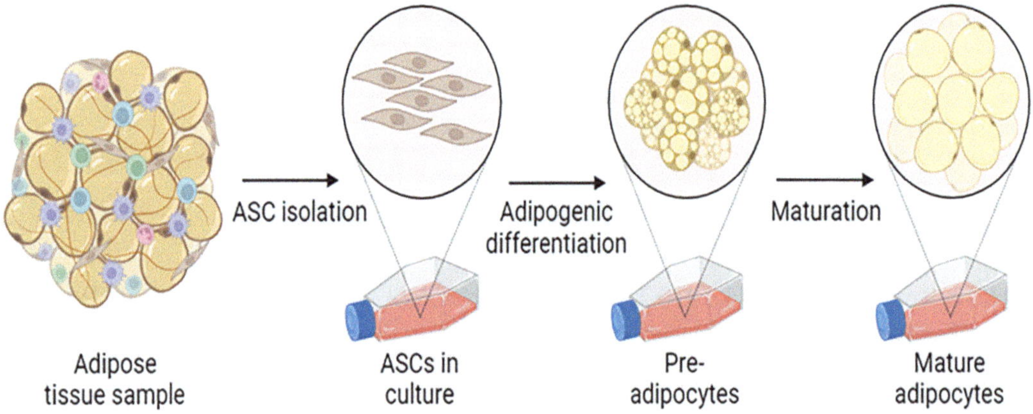


**Fig. 1** ASC isolation and adipogenic differentiation in vitro. Adipose-derived stromal/stem cells (ASCs) are isolated from adipose tissue and differentiated into mature adipocytes in vitro using adipocyte differentiation medium

lipid droplet quantities may, therefore, be used as important markers to determine onset or progression of disease [2]. Lipophilic staining dyes such as Nile Red are commercially available and can be used to visualize and quantify lipid droplets [8]. Nile Red is strongly fluorescent in a hydrophobic environment and has high binding affinity for neutral lipids, which are predominantly found in lipid droplet cores [8]. In this protocol, we provide a description on the quantification of lipid droplets in vitro using Nile Red staining.

## 2 Materials

### *2.1 Reagents*

1. Dulbecco's Modified Eagle's Medium (DMEM; with GlutaMAX™-I).
2. Penicillin (10,000 units/mL)–streptomycin (10,000 μg/mL) (Pen/Strep).
3. Fetal bovine serum (FBS).
4. 10 μg/mL human insulin.
5. 1 μM dexamethasone.
6. 200 μM indomethacin.
7. 0.5 M 3-isobutyl-methylxanthine.
8. 1× phosphate-buffered saline (PBS); pH ~ 7.4.
9. 2.5 μg/mL of 4′,6-diamino-2-phenylindole, dihydrochloride (DAPI).
10. 50 ng/mL of Nile Red in dimethyl sulfoxide (DMSO).

### 2.2 Equipment

1. Biosafety cabinet.
2. $CO_2$ incubator.
3. 6-well cell tissue culture plates.
4. Magnetic stirrer.
5. Vacuum aspirator.
6. Centrifuge.
7. Fluorescent microscope.

### 2.3 Medium Preparation

1. Complete growth medium (10% (v/v) FBS and 2% (v/v) Pen/Strep) (500 mL recipe): Measure 440 mL of Dulbecco's Modified Eagle Medium (DMEM; with GlutaMAX™-I). Add 50 mL of FBS, 10 mL of penicillin (10,000 units/mL)–streptomycin (10,000 μg/mL) (Pen/Strep). Store the media at ~4 °C until needed.
2. Adipogenic differentiation medium (500 mL recipe): Weigh out 55 mg of 3-isobutyl-methylxanthine and 35.8 mg of indomethacin, and add them to a sterile container in which you prepare the medium. Add 500 mL of complete growth medium, 1250 μL of human insulin and 100 μL of dexamethasone. Use a magnetic stirrer to mix the adipogenic differentiation medium at room temperature until all components have dissolved. Sterile filter the adipogenic differentiation solution. Store the media at ~4 °C until needed.

## 3 Method

### 3.1 Adipogenic Differentiation of ASCs

1. Seed ASCs at 5000 cells/cm$^2$ in 6-well plates, and culture in 2 mL of complete culture medium (*see* **Note 1**).
2. Incubate ASCs at 37 °C in 5% carbon dioxide ($CO_2$).
3. Grow cells to approximately 80–90% confluency, changing the complete culture medium twice a week (*see* **Note 2**).
4. Discard complete culture medium, and replace with adipogenic differentiation medium.
5. Grow cells in adipogenic differentiation medium for 21 days, changing the medium twice a week (*see* **Note 2**).

### 3.2 Staining of Adipocytes Following Differentiation

1. Add 1 μL of DAPI in each well and incubate overnight at 37 °C. (*see* **Note 3**)
2. Following the overnight step, add 10 μL of Nile Red into each well. (*see* **Note 3**)
3. Incubate cells at 37 °C for 20 min (*see* **Note 3**).
4. Wash cells twice with PBS to remove any unbound dye.

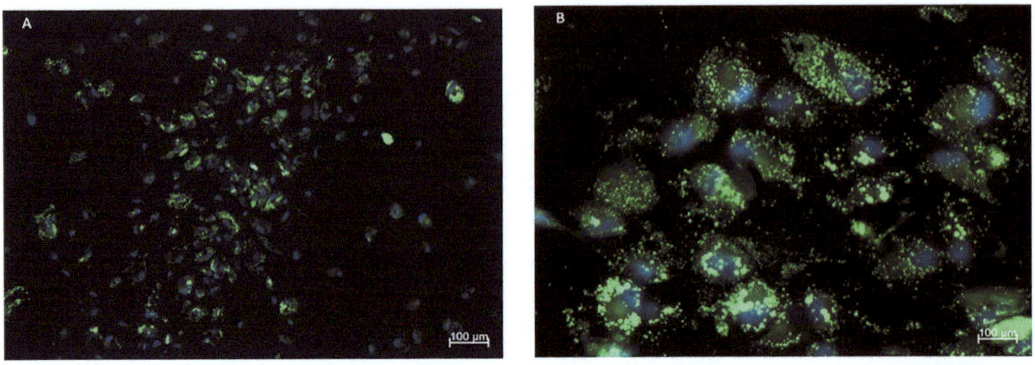


**Fig. 2** Microscopic images of differentiated adipocytes captured a 5× (**a**) and 20× (**b**) magnification

5. Add 1–2 mL of PBS into each well, and view cells under a fluorescent microscope (*see* **Note 4**).
6. Capture microscopic images at 20× for visualization of lipid droplets and at 5× magnification for quantification of the lipid droplets (Fig. 2).
7. Separate multicolor image to single color images representative of the two stains: DAPI (nuclei) and Nile Red (lipid droplets).

### *3.3 Semi-quantification of Lipid Droplets*

1. Download ImageJ Fiji software from the following link: https://imagej.nih.gov/ij/download.html.
2. Upload the lipid droplet (Nile Red stained) image to the software by selecting "File" and then "Open."
3. Convert the color image to grayscale by selecting "Image," "Type," and then "8-bit."
4. Convert the grayscale image to a binary image by selecting "Image," "Adjust," and "Threshold." (*see* **Note 5**)
5. Once the threshold settings have been established, select "Apply."
6. To analyze, select "Analyze" and then "Analyze Particles" using the default settings "Size: 0-Infinity" and "Circularity: 0.00–1.00", and then Select "OK."
7. To count, select "Analyze" and then "Measure."

## 4 Notes

1. Adipogenic differentiation experiments in this protocol were set up in 6-well plates.
2. The medium in the incubated cells must be replaced with fresh medium every 3 days.

3. Cells should be kept in the dark while staining to avoid loss of fluorescence.
4. Fluorescent microscopy should be conducted immediately after staining to avoid a decrease of fluorescent intensity of stained cells.
5. The threshold setting is important to separate pixels according to the object of interest from the background signal [9]. The threshold is manually selected between the minimum value of 0 and maximum value of 255, depending on the signal intensity. The threshold settings used were "Default" and "B&W" (black and white) colors.

## References

1. Fader Kaiser CM, Romano PS, Vanrell MC, Pocognoni CA, Jacob J, Caruso B, Delgui LR (2022) Biogenesis and breakdown of lipid droplets in pathological conditions. Front Cell Dev Biol 9. https://doi.org/10.3389/fcell.2021.826248
2. Zadoorian A, Du X, Yang H (2023) Lipid droplet biogenesis and functions in health and disease. Nat Rev Endocrinol 19:443–459. https://doi.org/10.1038/s41574-023-00845-0
3. Chen L, Jin Y, Wu J, Ren Z (2022) Lipid droplets: a cellular organelle vital for thermogenesis. Int J Biol Sci 18:6176–6188. https://doi.org/10.7150/ijbs.77051
4. Yang H, Liu J (2021) Chapter 11 – structure and function of lipid droplets. In: Ridgway ND, McLeod RS (eds) Biochemistry of lipids, lipoproteins and membranes, 7th edn. Elsevier, London, pp 357–394
5. Heid H, Rickelt S, Zimbelmann R, Winter S, Schumacher H, Dörflinger Y, Kuhn C, Franke WW (2014) On the formation of lipid droplets in human adipocytes: the organization of the perilipin-vimentin cortex. PLoS One 9:e90386. https://doi.org/10.1371/journal.pone.0090386
6. Tsuji W, Rubin JP, Marra KG (2014) Adipose-derived stem cells: implications in tissue regeneration. World J Stem Cells 6:312–321. https://doi.org/10.4252/wjsc.v6.i3.312
7. Blücher C, Stadler SC (2017) Obesity and breast cancer: current insights on the role of fatty acids and lipid metabolism in promoting breast cancer growth and progression. Front Endocrinol 8. https://doi.org/10.3389/fendo.2017.00293
8. Martinez V, Henary M (2016) Nile red and nile blue: applications and syntheses of structural analogues. Chemistry 22:13764–13782. https://doi.org/10.1002/chem.201601570
9. Rasband WS (1997–2018) ImageJ. U.-S. National Institutes of Health Bethesda, Maryland

Chapter 6

# RT-qPCR Quantification of Adipogenic Marker Genes (PPARg, C/EBPa, FABP4, and CD36)

Carina C. Babbo, Reabetswe R. Pitere, Rachel Giles, Melvin A. Ambele, and Michael S. Pepper

## Abstract

Adipogenesis is a complex multiphase process in which preadipocytes develop into adipocytes. This tightly regulated process is facilitated by a cascade of genes and transcription factors. In this chapter, we describe a protocol that can be used to quantify the expression of adipogenic markers using RT-qPCR.

**Key words** RT-qPCR, adipogenesis, PPARg, C/EBPa, FABP4, CD36

## 1 Introduction

Adipose tissue is regarded as a metabolic organ and functions as an endocrine organ and caloric reservoir. Adipose tissue plays an important role in the production and secretion of various factors such as lipids, adipokines, and fatty acids, which regulate energy metabolism [1, 2]. Adipose tissue is primarily composed of adipocytes and the process by which new adipocytes are formed is known as adipogenesis [2].

Adipogenesis is a complex multistep process in which mesenchymal precursor cells undergo commitment to become adipocyte precursor cells (preadipocytes), which eventually differentiate into mature adipocytes [3]. During each phase of adipogenesis, the sequential activation and/or inhibition of specific transcription factors drive differentiation and ensure preadipocytes are differentiated into mature and functional adipocytes [2, 3]. Among these transcription factors are peroxisome proliferator-activated receptor gamma (PPARg) and CCAAT/enhancer binding protein alpha (C/EBPa), which are critical in adipogenesis. C/EBPa promotes the expression of PPARg, which is the key regulator of adipogenesis [4]. The lack of PPARY expression results in the precursor cells not

Michael S. Pepper and Melvin A. Ambele (eds.), *Adipogenesis: Methods and Protocols*, Methods in Molecular Biology, vol. 2938, https://doi.org/10.1007/978-1-0716-4607-6_6,

displaying the adipocyte phenotype [3, 4]. There are two isoforms of the PPARg transcription factor, namely, PPARg1 and PPARg2, which arise through alternative promoter usage. The PPARg1 isoform can be found in all cells, but PPARg2 is restricted to adipose tissue and is considered a better transcription activator of adipogenesis [5, 6]. Apart from PPARg and C/EBPa, various other genes have been shown to play an active role in producing the mature adipocyte [3, 7, 8]. PPARg and C/EBPα regulate the expression of fatty acid-binding protein 4 (*FABP4*), which interacts with cluster of differentiation 36 (CD36) to promote fatty acid transport and metabolism during adipogenesis [9, 10].

In this chapter, we will describe the use of real-time quantitative PCR (RT-qPCR) to study the expression of PPARg, C/EBPa, FABP4, and CD36 during adipogenesis. RT-qPCR combines reverse transcription, PCR amplification, and fluorescence to investigate gene expression. First, RNA is used as a template for complementary DNA (cDNA) synthesis using reverse transcription enzymes. The cDNA is then used as product for the amplification reaction. The amount of template increases exponentially with every amplification cycle, which is monitored using fluorescence. There are different ways to monitor fluorescence, but we will focus on SYBR Green, which is a double-stranded DNA (dsDNA) intercalating dye that binds to the minor grooves of DNA. Initially, the dye emits very low levels of fluorescence, which then exponentially increase as the cDNA is amplified and the amount of dsDNA increases (Fig. 1A) [11–13]. The point at which the signal exceeds the background signal is called the threshold cycle ($C_T$) or crossing point (Cp) (Fig. 1B, point b). The more initial target template available, the fewer cycles will be required in order to cross the threshold [13, 14]. Eventually, the signal will cease to increase, and a plateau phase will be reached due to the exhaustion of primers and dNTP availability for incorporation (Fig. 1, point d).

Using this method, gene expression can be quantified into two ways—absolute or relative quantification. Absolute quantification makes use of a set of standards at different concentrations where the initial copy number of the target gene is known. These standards are used to make a standard curve to which the Cp value of the sample in question is compared to. Relative quantification, on the other hand, does not require the use of standard curves. Gene expression is calculated relative to a reference gene, calibrator, and an untreated or time 0 sample using mathematical equations illustrated in Equation 1 and Fig. 2 [13, 14]. The most often used method to calculate relative gene expression is the delta–delta Ct method, i.e., $2 - \Delta\Delta CT$. However, this method assumes a qPCR efficiency of 100%, which is not necessarily always true. Rao and colleagues [15] have shown that this method can be improved by using the amplification efficiency (E) of each gene of interest, altering the formula to $E^{-\Delta\Delta CT}$ (Equation 2). The amplification

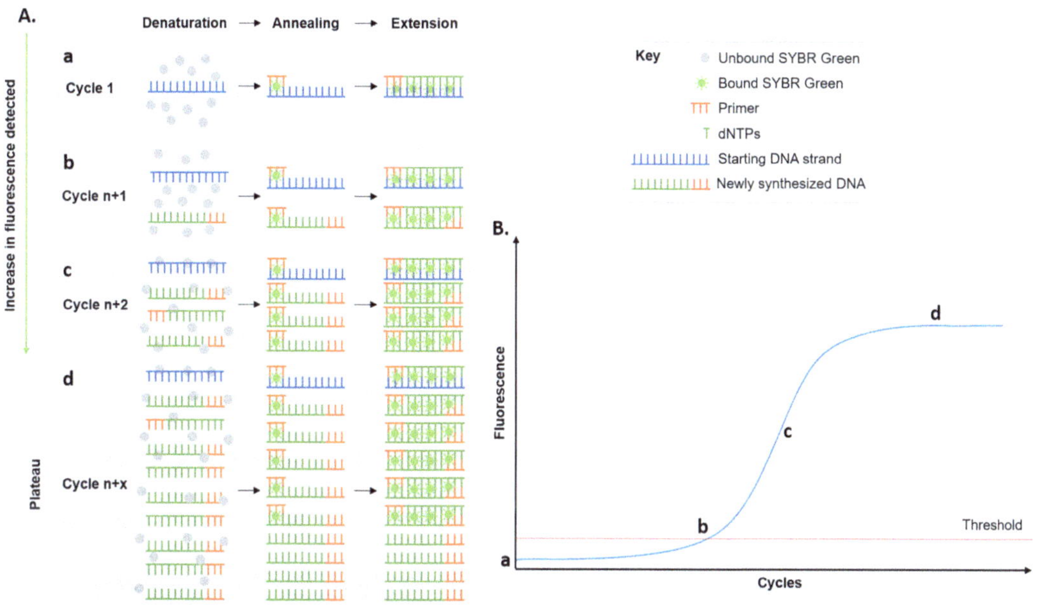


**Fig. 1** SYBR Green RT-qPCR principles. SYBR Green is a double-stranded DNA intercalating dye. The dye emits a stronger fluorescence signal when bound to double-stranded DNA than when unbound in solution (background) (**A**-a; red line in **B**). The point at which the amplification-associated fluorescence signal intercepts the background fluorescence is known as the threshold cycle (CT), shown as point b in **B**. As the amplification cycles continue, the amount of double-stranded DNA and thus signal detected will increase exponentially (**B**-c) until reaching a plateau (**B**-d)

efficiency is determined with the aid of a standard curve (Equation 3). An amplification efficiency of 1 is desired as it is an indication that the product to be amplified is doubling with every cycle. Efficiencies above 1 may be attributed to contaminant carry over from either the RNA isolation step (ethanol, phenol) or cDNA synthesis (reverse transcriptase).

## Equation 1: Calculating ΔΔCt

*Step 1: Calculate the difference between the target and reference gene for the induced (treated) group (ΔCT):*

$$\Delta CT = (CT\ Target\ gene - CT\ Reference\ gene)\,Induced \quad (1.1)$$

*Step 2: Calculate the difference between the target and reference gene for the non-induced (control) group (ΔCT):*

$$\Delta CT = (CT\ Target\ gene - CT\ Reference\ gene)\,Non\text{-}induced \quad (1.2)$$

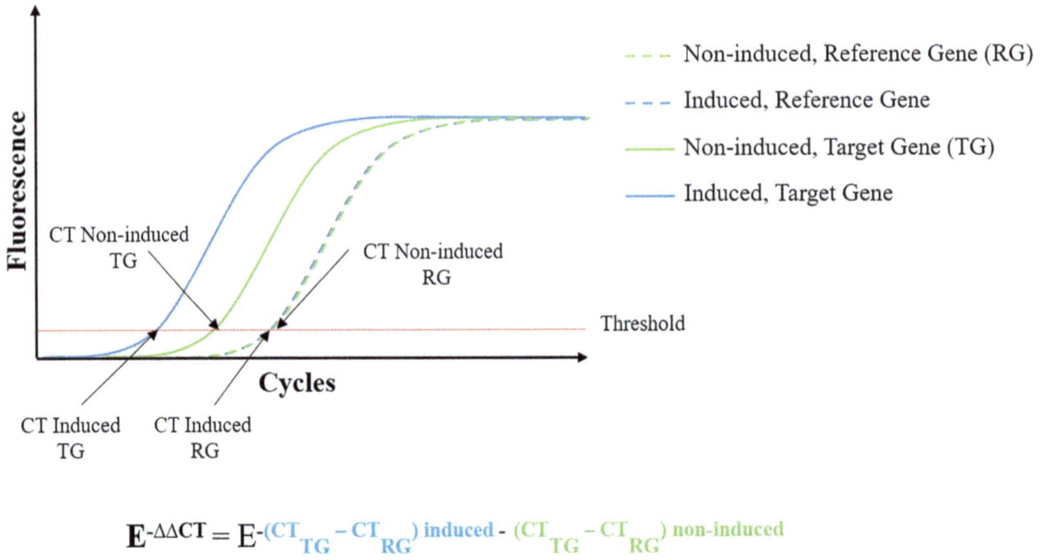


**Fig. 2** Schematic Illustration of the Mathematical Basis of Relative Quantification by RT-qPCR, modified from VanGuilder et al. (2015). Using the relative quantification method for quantitation in RT-qPCR, the expression of a target gene in the test sample is measured relative to a control sample (e.g., untreated sample), calibrator, or reference gene. In the illustration above, non-induced represents the untreated sample and induced represents the treated sample. Note that the induced sample crosses the threshold before the non-induced sample. This indicates that the treatment (induction) resulted in the upregulation of the target gene. Also note that the reference gene has the same Ct value under both non-induced and induced conditions. Ideally, the expression of the reference/control gene should not change under treatment conditions

***Step 3: Calculate the difference between the two groups (ΔΔCT):***

$$\Delta\Delta CT = (\Delta CT)\, Induced - (\Delta CT)\, Non\text{-}induced \tag{1.3}$$

**Equation 2: Modified ΔΔCt**

$$E^{-\Delta\Delta CT}$$

**Equation 3: Amplification Efficiency**

$$E = 10 \times \frac{-1}{S} - 1$$

$S =$ *Slope of the standard curve*

## 2 Materials

### 2.1 Reagents

1. Complete growth medium: Add 50 mL of FBS and 10 mL of penicillin (10,000 units/mL)–streptomycin (10,000 μg/mL) (Pen/Strep) to 440 mL of Dulbecco's Modified Eagle Medium (DMEM; with GlutaMAX™-I). Store the media at between 4 and 8 °C.

**Table 1**
**Primer pairs for adipogenic genes**

| Gene | Forward primer (3′ to 5′) | Reverse Primer (3′ to 5′) |
|---|---|---|
| PPARY | CGTGGATCTCTCCGTAAT | TGGATCTGTTCTTGTGAATG |
| C/EBPα | GTCTCTGCTAAACCACCA | AAAGGAAAGGGAGTCTCAG |
| FABP4 | ATCAACCACCATAAAGAGAAA | AACTTCAGTCCAGGTCAA |
| CD36 | CTTTGCCTCTCCAGTTGAA | ACACAGGTCTCCCTTCTT |

**Table 2**
**Primer pairs for reference genes**

| Gene | Forward primer (3′ to 5′) | Reverse Primer (3′ to 5′) |
|---|---|---|
| *PPIA* | GAGTTAAGAGTGTTGATGTAGG | CCTGGGACTGGAAAGTAA |
| *TBP* | CCGAAACGCCGAATATAA | GGACTGTTCTTCACTCTTG |
| *YWHAZ* | TGACATTGGGTAGCATTAAC | GCACCTGACAAATAGAAAGA |

2. Adipogenic differentiation medium: Weigh out 55 mg of 3-isobutyl-methylxanthine (0.5 M) and 35.8 mg of indomethacin (200 μM). Add 500 mL complete growth medium, 1250 μL of human insulin (10 μg/mL), and 100 μL of dexamethasone (1 μM). Use a magnetic stirrer to mix the adipogenic differentiation medium at room temperature until all components have dissolved. Store at 4 °C.
3. Phosphate-buffered saline (PBS; pH 7.4). Store it at −20 °C.
4. Primer pairs for adipogenesis genes(Table 1) and reference genes [16] (Table 2). Store primers at −20 °C.

### 2.2 Equipment

1. 5% $CO_2$/37°C water-jacked incubator.
2. Culture flaks.
3. Pipettes.
4. Magnetic stirrer.
5. Scale.
6. Vortex mixer.
7. NanoDrop® ND 1000 spectrophotometer or other equivalent.
8. TapeStation® 2200 platform (Agilent Technologies) or other equivalent.
9. RT-qPCR machine.

### 2.3 Kits

1. Qiagen RNeasy Mini Kit.
2. SensiFAST™ cDNA synthesis kit.
3. RT-qPCR SYBR Green kit.

## 3 Methods

### 3.1 Adipogenic Differentiation of ASCs

1. Seed ASCs at a density of 5000 cells/cm$^2$ in T80 flasks and culture in 7 mL of complete culture medium. In order to have control cells (non-induced), plate 2× T80 flasks. Use one flask for induced cells and the other flask for non-induced cells (control).
2. Incubate ASCs at 37°C in 5% carbon dioxide ($CO_2$). Replace the culture medium with fresh medium twice a week.
3. Grow cells to approximately 80% confluency.
4. Discard the complete culture medium from the plate in which you wish to differentiate the cells in.
5. Add 7 mL of adipogenic differentiation medium to cells you want to differentiate in flask.
6. Continue to grow the control cells (non-induced) in complete culture medium.
7. Allow the induced cells to grow and differentiate for 21 days in parallel with the non-induced (control) cells, and change the respective medium in the flask every 3–4 days.

### 3.2 Trypsinization of Cells

1. Aspirate medium from cells.
2. Add 7 mL of PBS to each flask to wash any remaining medium.
3. Add 4 mL of 0.25% trypsin-EDTA to the cells, and incubate for approximately 7 min at 37 °C to make sure cells completely dislodged from the flask surface into a suspension.
4. Add an equivalent volume of complete culture medium (4 mL) to trypsin-EDTA in cells to stop the action of trypsin on cells.
5. Label two 15 mL centrifuge tubes as follows:
   (a) Non-induced cells (control).
   (b) Induced cells.
6. Transfer the cell suspension into the relevant 15 mL centrifuge tube.
7. Top up the tubes with PBS to a volume of between 10 mL and 14 mL to wash the cells.
8. Centrifuge the cell suspension at 300× *g* for 5 min.
9. Repeat the wash step two more times to remove any remaining phenol red from the medium.

10. Aspirate the PBS and leave the cell pellet undisturbed.
11. Resuspend the cells in 1 mL of PBS.
12. Transfer the cell suspensions into a 1.5 mL Eppendorf tube, and centrifuge at 500× *g* for 5 min.
13. The cells are now ready for RNA extraction using an RNA extraction kit of choice (*see* **Note 2**).

### 3.3 RNA Integrity

The integrity of isolated RNA can further be determined on a TapeStation® 2200 platform (Agilent Technologies; Santa Clara, CA, USA) using the RNA Screen Tape® (Agilent Technologies; Santa Clara, CA, USA) and sample buffer (Agilent Technologies; Santa Clara, CA, USA).

1. Add 5 μL of sample buffer to 1 μL of RNA (RNA concentration can range between 25 and 500 ng/μL).
2. Vortex sample for 1 min to ensure thorough mixing.
3. Transfer sample to a thermocycler to be heated to 72 °C for 3 min.
4. Place the sample on ice for 2 min.
5. Analyze the sample using the RNA Screen Tape® on the TapeStation® 2200. A RINe value ≥8 is indicative of intact high-quality RNA (Fig. 3).

### 3.4 cDNA Synthesis

cDNA synthesis can be done using the SensiFAST™ cDNA synthesis kit according to the manufacturer's instructions:

1. Add 1 μg of RNA to the master mix:

| | Volumes (μL) for 1× reaction | |
|---|---|---|
| **Reaction component** | **Samples** | **Control[a]** |
| 5× TransAmp buffer | 4 | 4 |
| Reverse transcriptase | 1 | 0[a] |
| 1 μg RNA[a] | Variable | Variable |
| Nuclease-free water | Variable | Variable |
| **Final reaction volume** | **20 μL** | **20 μL** |

[a]Preparing a no reverse transcriptase control will help determine whether there is any genomic DNA contamination in your samples

2. Gently mix by pipetting up and down.
3. Run sample on a thermocycler using the following setup:
   (i) Priming at 25 °C for 10 min.
   (ii) Reverse transcription at 42 °C for 15 min.

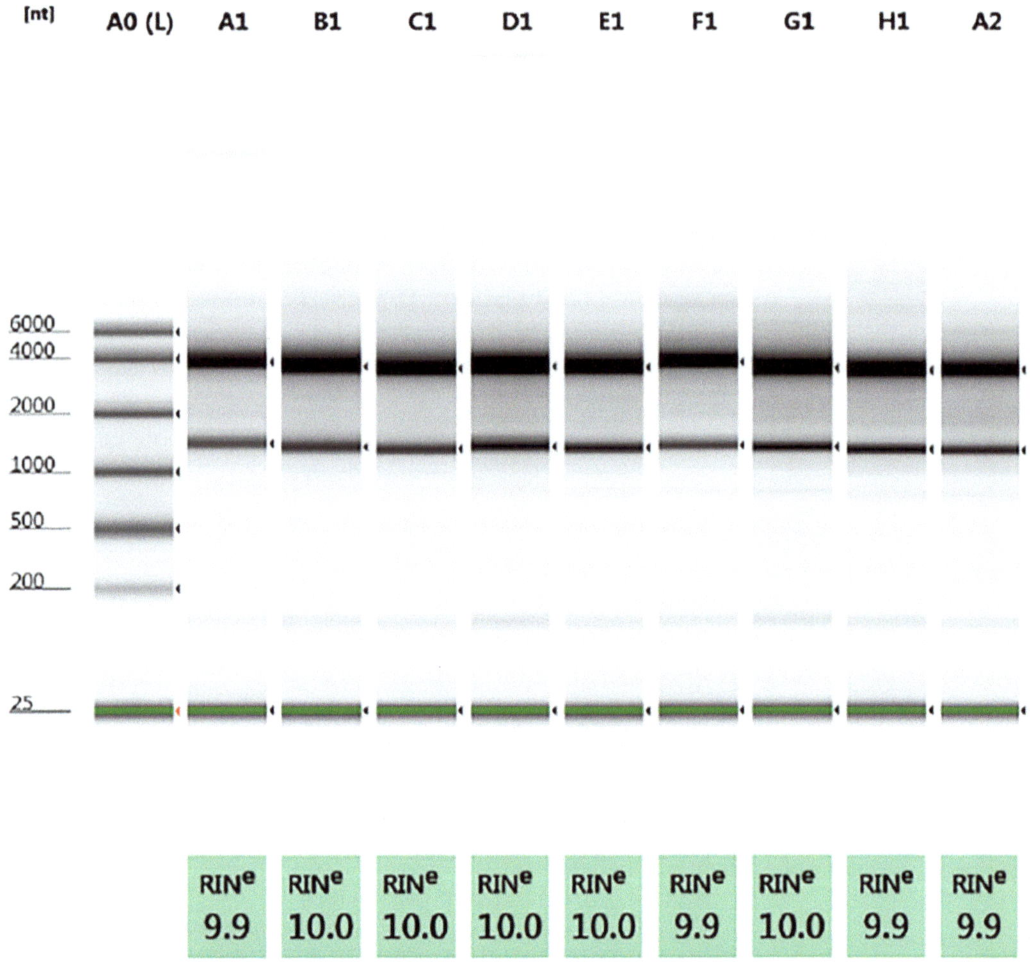


**Fig. 3** Representative image of RNA integrity results obtained from TapeStation® 2200. Lane "A0" represents the ladder; remaining lanes (A1–A2) represent the samples tested. The green blocks beneath the lanes represent the test results i.e. RIN$^e$ values

(iii) RT inactivation at 85 °C for 5 min.

(iv) Hold at 4 °C for infinity.

4. Measure the cDNA concentration and quality (A260/A280) using a NanoDrop® ND 1000 spectrophotometer (*see* **Note 4**).
5. Use ~20 ng/uL of synthesized cDNA for RT-qPCR.
6. The cDNA can be stored at −20 °C until used in RT-qPCR experiments.

### 3.5 RT-qPCR

There are many available kits on the market for RT-qPCR. Here, we will make use of the LightCycler® 480 SYBR Green Master Mix Kit.

1. Prepare the RT-qPCR reaction setup for LightCycler® 480 SYBR Green I Master Mix for amplification as per manufacturer's instructions as follows:

| Reagent | Quantity for 1 reaction | Volume for 1 reaction (μL) |
|---|---|---|
| SYBR green master mix | 1× | 5 |
| Forward primer | 400 nM | 0.4 |
| Reverse primer | 400 nM | 0.4 |
| cDNA template (25 ng/μL) | – | 2 |
| PCR grade water | – | 2.2 |
| Total volume | – | 10 μL |

2. RT-qPCR cycle conditions.

| PCR condition | Temperature (°C) | Duration | Number of cycles |
|---|---|---|---|
| Initial denaturation | 95 | 5 min | 1 |
| Denaturation<br>Extension<br>Annealing | 95<br>62<br>62 | 30 s<br>30 s<br>30 s | 40 |

## 4 Notes

1. Medium must be changed every 3 days in the cultured cells.
2. Make sure the kit you use is appropriate for the number of cells you are extracting RNA from. A cell count may need to be determined prior to RNA extraction. If you have too many cells ($> 2 \times 10^6$), simply split them so that you are using the appropriate number of cells for your kit.
3. The A260/A280 ratio of ~1.8 is generally accepted as pure for DNA, and a A260/A280 ratio of ~2.0 is generally accepted as pure for RNA. A A260/A280 ratio outside the recommended range is suggestive of contaminants in the sample.
4. All qPCR reactions must be set up in a laminar flow cabinet to prevent contamination.

## References


1. Frühbeck G, Catalán V, Rodríguez A, Gómez-Ambrosi J (2018) Adiponectin-leptin ratio: a promising index to estimate adipose tissue dysfunction. Relation with obesity-associated cardiometabolic risk. Adipocytes 7:57–62. https://doi.org/10.1080/21623945.2017.1402151
2. Audano M, Pedretti S, Caruso D, Crestani M, De Fabiani E, Mitro N (2022) Regulatory mechanisms of the early phase of white adipocyte differentiation: an overview. Cell Mol Life Sci 79:139. https://doi.org/10.1007/s00018-022-04169-6
3. Ghaben AL, Scherer PE (2019) Adipogenesis and metabolic health. Nat Rev Mol Cell Biol 20:242–258. https://doi.org/10.1038/s41580-018-0093-z
4. Rosen ED, Hsu CH, Wang X, Sakai S, Freeman MW, Gonzalez FJ, Spiegelman BM (2002) C/EBPalpha induces adipogenesis through PPARgamma: a unified pathway. Genes Dev 16:22–26. https://doi.org/10.1101/gad.948702
5. Rosen ED, Walkey CJ, Puigserver P, Spiegelman BM (2000) Transcriptional regulation of adipogenesis. Genes Dev 14:1293–1307
6. Janani C, Ranjitha Kumari BD (2015) PPAR gamma gene – a review. Diabetes Metab Syndr 9:46–50. https://doi.org/10.1016/j.dsx.2014.09.015
7. Longo M, Zatterale F, Naderi J, Parrillo L, Formisano P, Raciti GA, Beguinot F, Miele C (2019) Adipose tissue dysfunction as determinant of obesity-associated metabolic complications. Int J Mol Sci 20:2358
8. Ambele MA, Dhanraj P, Giles R, Pepper MS (2020) Adipogenesis: a complex interplay of multiple molecular determinants and pathways. Int J Mol Sci 21. https://doi.org/10.3390/ijms21124283
9. Gyamfi J, Yeo JH, Kwon D, Min BS, Cha YJ, Koo JS, Jeong J, Lee J, Choi J (2021) Interaction between CD36 and FABP4 modulates adipocyte-induced fatty acid import and metabolism in breast cancer. NPJ Breast Cancer 7:129. https://doi.org/10.1038/s41523-021-00324-7
10. Trojnar M, Patro-Małysza J, Kimber-Trojnar Ż, Leszczyńska-Gorzelak B, Mosiewicz J (2019) Associations between fatty acid-binding protein 4–A proinflammatory adipokine and insulin resistance, gestational and type 2 diabetes mellitus. Cells 8:227
11. Valasek MA, Repa JJ (2005) The power of real-time PCR. Adv Physiol Educ 29:151–159. https://doi.org/10.1152/advan.00019.2005
12. Cao H, Shockey JM (2012) Comparison of TaqMan and SYBR green qPCR methods for quantitative gene expression in tung tree tissues. J Agric Food Chem 60:12296–12303. https://doi.org/10.1021/jf304690e
13. VanGuilder HD, Vrana KE, Freeman WM (2008) Twenty-five years of quantitative PCR for gene expression analysis. BioTechniques 44:619–626. https://doi.org/10.2144/000112776
14. Arya M, Shergill IS, Williamson M, Gommersall L, Arya N, Patel HR (2005) Basic principles of real-time quantitative PCR. Expert Rev Mol Diagn 5:209–219. https://doi.org/10.1586/14737159.5.2.209
15. Rao X, Huang X, Zhou Z, Lin X (2013) An improvement of the 2^(-delta delta CT) method for quantitative real-time polymerase chain reaction data analysis. Biostat Bioinforma Biomath 3:71–85
16. Ambele MA, Dessels C, Durandt C, Pepper MS (2016) Genome-wide analysis of gene expression during adipogenesis in human adipose-derived stromal cells reveals novel patterns of gene expression during adipocyte differentiation. Stem Cell Res 16:725–734

# Chapter 7

# Adipogenic Differentiation of Human Adipose-Derived Mesenchymal Stromal/Stem Cells (ASCs)

**Ladislaus Tapiwa Adam, Reabetswe R. Pitere, Melvin A. Ambele, and Michael S. Pepper**

## Abstract

Adipose-derived stromal/stem cells (ASCs) from human fat tissue samples offer a valuable model to study adipogenesis in vitro. A hormonal cocktail that promotes growth and differentiation can be used in experimental procedures to facilitate the conversion of ASCs into adipocytes. This protocol describes methods for adipogenic differentiation of primary human ASCs in vitro, outlining flow cytometry quantification and fluorescence microscopy qualitative assessment of the adipogenic process.

**Key words** Adipose-derived stromal/stem cells, Adipogenesis, Adipogenic differentiation, Flow cytometry, Fluorescence microscopy, 3-Isobutyl-methylxanthine, Indomethacin, Rosiglitazone

## 1 Introduction

Adipose-derived stromal/stem cells (ASCs) are widely accepted as the cells of origin of adipocytes, and these precursor cells are considered to originate from mesenchymal stromal/stem cells (MSCs) [1, 2]. Stem cells hold great promise in regenerative medicine for use as cell-based therapies mainly owing to their self-renewal and multilineage differentiation potential [2]. In vitro, a combination of hormones in the form of a cocktail termed MDI is commonly used to induce differentiation. This cocktail consists of M, 3-isobutyl-1-methylxanthine (IBMX); D, dexamethasone; and I, insulin. IBMX acts as a phosphodiesterase inhibitor enhancing adipogenesis by promoting the expression of CCAAT/enhancer-binding protein (C/EBPβ) through cAMP response element binding protein [3]. Dexamethasone, a glucocorticoid, stimulates adipogenesis through direct induction of genes responsible for C/EBPβ and C/EBPδ expression [4, 5]. Insulin promotes glucose uptake into cells, which is then stored as triacyglycerols, and plays a role in activating proliferation and differentiation of

Michael S. Pepper and Melvin A. Ambele (eds.), *Adipogenesis: Methods and Protocols*, Methods in Molecular Biology, vol. 2938, https://doi.org/10.1007/978-1-0716-4607-6_7,

preadipocytes [4]. Sometimes, MDI is supplemented with indomethacin (cyclooxygenase inhibitor) and rosiglitazone (PPARγ agonist), which help to induce adipogenesis by stimulating PPARγ expression and transcriptional activity, respectively [6]. This chapter describes the procedure for differentiating primary human ASCs in vitro and highlights flow cytometric and fluorescent microscopy assessments to assess adipogenesis.

## 2 Materials

### 2.1 Adipose-Derived Stromal/Stem Cells

Human adipose-derived stromal/stem cells (ASCs) can be used either as freshly isolated or cryopreserved. ASCs can be isolated from either lipoaspirates or solid fat tissue samples. ASCs can also be expanded to increase cell numbers before adipogenic differentiation.

### 2.2 Equipment

1. Laminar air flow cabinet (BSL II).
2. $CO_2$ incubator.
3. Centrifuge.
4. Vacuum aspirator.
5. Magnetic stirrer and bars.
6. Inverted microscope.
7. Flow cytometer.
8. Fluorescence microscope.

### 2.3 General Materials and Supplies

1. Tissue culture plates and flasks (*see* **Note 1**).
2. Pipettes and pipette tips.
3. Centrifuge tubes.
4. Filter units (0.22 μm).

### 2.4 Reagents

1. Complete DMEM medium (*see* **Note 2**): Add 50 mL of fetal bovine serum (10% vol/vol) and 10 mL of Pen/Strep (2% vol/vol) to 440 mL of DMEM medium. Gently invert the bottle a few times to ensure proper mixing, and store the media at 2–8 °C.
2. Adipogenic induction medium (500 mL): Weigh out 55 mg of 3-isobutyl-methylxanthine (0.5 M final concentration), 35.8 mg of indomethacin (200 μM final concentration), 1250 μL of insulin (10 μg/mL final concentration), and 100 μL of dexamethasone (5 μM final concentration) (*see* **Note 3**), and add to 500 mL of complete DMEM in a glass bottle. Place a sterile magnetic stirrer bar inside the bottle, and stir the solution overnight (12–18 h) at room temperature on the magnetic stirrer. Filter the medium using a 0.22 μm sterile filter, and then label and store it at 2–8 °C.

## 3 Methods

### 3.1 Adipogenic Differentiation

1. Seed ASCs at a density of 5000 cells/cm$^2$, and maintain cells in complete DMEM medium under normal culture conditions (37 °C/5% $CO_2$) until 90–100% confluent. Change medium after every 3–4 days (*see* **Note 4**).
2. On reaching 90–100% confluency, aspirate the medium and discard; then, add 2 mL of adipogenic induction medium, and maintain cells in this medium.
3. Replace adipogenic induction medium once every 2 days for 21 days (*see* **Note 5**).

### 3.2 Flow Cytometric Adipogenic Quantification (see Note 6)

When differentiation is complete, trypsinize the cells as follows:

1. Aspirate the adipogenic induction medium; then, add 500 μL of trypsin-EDTA to cells, and incubate for about 7–10 min.
2. Check if the cells have dislodged from the bottom of the flask into a cell suspension (*see* **Note 7**); once dislodged, add 500 μL of complete DMEM medium to neutralize/stop the activity of trypsin.
3. Transfer 1 mL of the cell suspension into separate tubes.
4. Stain the cell suspension with Nile Red and DAPI stain to a final concentration of 0.02 μg/mL and 5 ng/mL, respectively (*see* **Note 8**).
5. Incubate at 37 °C for 30 min followed by flow cytometric analysis immediately (*see* Chap. 2).

### 3.3 Fluorescence Microscopy Staining Procedure

1. Aspirate adipogenic induction medium from wells, and replace with fresh complete medium (*see* **Note 9**).
2. Stain ASCs with a final concentration of 0.1 μg/mL of Nile Red stain and 2.5 μM VDC violet.
3. Incubate for 20 min at 37 °C, 5% $CO_2$.
4. Aspirate the medium, followed by washing twice with phosphate-buffered saline (PBS); pH ~ 7.4.
5. Add 1 mL of PBS to each well.
6. Capture fluorescence images under a microscope (*see* Chap. 5).

## 4 Notes

1. Adipogenesis experiments described here were performed in 6-well plates. Twelve-well plates are also suitable especially for experiments where high cell numbers are not required. There were no significant differences in adipogenic differentiation

observed between cells cultured in 6-well and 12-well plates. However, cell clumping was noted in the middle of wells particularly when seeding cells in 6-well plates. It is recommended to move the plate on a flat surface in a figure eight pattern; however, the following plating strategy gave better results: add 1 mL medium to 6-well plates (ensure medium covers well surface), followed by the addition of 1 mL cell suspension. Gently move the plate back and forth and then side to side. Leave the plate to stand on a flat surface (away from vibrations/motion) for 30 min before final incubation. Pipetting the cell suspension up and down before moving the flask into the incubator will reduce the formation of cell clumps. Importantly, avoid swirling of plate during seeding as this increases the chances of cell clumping, although adipogenic differentiation was unaffected with cell clumping in the middle of the well.

2. DMEM without pyruvate and without phenol red was used in our experiments, and adipogenic differentiation was not affected. This is because phenol red interferes with florescence and flow cytometry measurements [9]. DMEM with pyruvate is also suitable and has been used for adipogenic differentiation in our laboratory.
3. In other experiments in our laboratory, dexamethasone to a final concentration of 1 μM has been used for differentiation with good results.
4. Preincubate medium from the fridge for at least 1 h at 37 °C before introducing to cells; this prevents cell shock due to the wide temperature difference.
5. Care should be taken not to disturb the cells when aspirating medium, as adipocytes are fragile and tend to detach easily from the flask surface. Regular checks of cultures for contamination and yellowing of medium are recommended to ensure cell vitality and viability are maintained.
6. Adipogenic differentiation of human ASCs was better at passages below 5 (P5); in other cultures, passages below P7 also gave satisfactory ACS differentiation capacity. However, an increase in cell passage numbers of between P10 and P14 showed a significant decrease in adipogenic differentiation capacity of the cells [7].
7. If cells do not dislodge, give the plate a gentle shake, and make sure trypsin-EDTA has covered the entire surface of the flask (add more trypsin-EDTA if necessary) and has not evaporated. Also, if cells have not dislodged, increase the incubation time, 2 min at a time until cells dislodge, and make a note of this. Be gentle when handling cells as adipocytes are fragile, and it is advisable to minimize additional wash steps to prevent the

release of intracellular lipid droplets from differentiated adipocytes. Use pipette tips with a wide bore or disposable Pasteur pipettes for cell suspension transfers.

8. Nile Red stain is our preferred dye used to stain lipid droplets instead of Oil Red O stain because Oil Red O is relatively cell impermeable and does not penetrate live cells; the dye is also nonfluorescent and therefore unsuitable for flow cytometry [8].
9. Alternatively, use PBS supplemented with 10% fetal bovine serum.

## References


1. Vishvanath L, Long JZ, Spiegelman BM, Gupta RK (2017) Do adipocytes emerge from mural progenitors? Cell Stem Cell 20:585–586. https://doi.org/10.1016/j.stem.2017.03.013
2. Si Z, Wang X, Sun C et al (2019) Adipose-derived stem cells: sources, potency, and implications for regenerative therapies. Biomed Pharmacother 114:108765. https://doi.org/10.1016/J.BIOPHA.2019.108765
3. Lee M-J (2017) Hormonal regulation of adipogenesis. Compr Physiol 7:1151–1195. https://doi.org/10.1002/cphy.c160047
4. Moseti D, Regassa A, Kim WK (2016) Molecular regulation of adipogenesis and potential anti-adipogenic bioactive molecules. Int J Mol Sci 17:1–24. https://doi.org/10.3390/ijms17010124
5. Scott MA, Nguyen VT, Levi B, James AW (2011) Current methods of adipogenic differentiation of mesenchymal stem cells. Stem Cells Dev 20:1793–1804. https://doi.org/10.1089/scd.2011.0040
6. Saben J, Thakali KM, Lindsey FE et al (2014) Distinct adipogenic differentiation phenotypes of human umbilical cord mesenchymal cells dependent on adipogenic conditions. Exp Biol Med 239:1340–1351. https://doi.org/10.1177/1535370214539225
7. Safwani WKZW, Makpol S, Sathapan S, Chua K (2014) Impact of adipogenic differentiation on stemness and osteogenic gene expression in extensive culture of human adipose-derived stem cells. Arch Med Sci 10:597–606. https://doi.org/10.5114/aoms.2014.43753
8. Boumelhem BB, Assinder SJ, Bell-Anderson KS, Fraser ST (2017) Flow cytometric single cell analysis reveals heterogeneity between adipose depots. Adipocytes 6:112–123. https://doi.org/10.1080/21623945.2017.1319536
9. Wu D, Yotnda P (2011) Production and detection of Reactive Oxygen Species (ROS) in cancers. J Vis Exp:e3357. https://doi.org/10.3791/3357

# Chapter 8

# Western Blot Detection of Adipogenic Protein


## Pontsho Moela



## Abstract

Western blotting (WB) is an end-point technique that is used to analyze the expression of target proteins in cells and tissues. It involves the separation of proteins using SDS-PAGE followed by an electrophoretic transfer of the proteins from the gel to a hydrophobic membrane where they will be immunodetected and captured on a film or by an imager. The peroxisome proliferator-activated receptor gamma (PPARγ) is a type of nuclear receptor protein that plays a crucial role in regulating gene expression and various cellular functions. In this chapter, the western blot procedure is demonstrated for the detection and quantification of the PPARγ nuclear protein from either adipocyte cell lines or adipose tissue.



**Key words** Western blot, Chemiluminescence, SDS-PAGE, Lipid metabolism, PPARγ


## 1 Introduction

Western blotting (WB) is an end-point technique that is used to analyze the expression of target proteins in cells and tissues [1]. It involves the separation of proteins using SDS-PAGE followed by an electrophoretic transfer of the proteins from the gel to a hydrophobic membrane where they will be immunodetected and captured on a film or by an imager [2].

The peroxisome proliferator-activated receptor gamma (PPARγ) is the master regulator of adipogenesis and plays a crucial role in regulating gene expression and various cellular functions [3, 4]. PPARγ is primarily associated with adipocyte (fat cell) differentiation and lipid metabolism. It is a member of the nuclear hormone receptor superfamily and acts as a transcription factor, influencing the expression of genes involved in glucose homeostasis, lipid metabolism, and inflammation [5].

PPARγ is particularly important in the regulation of adipogenesis, which is the process by which undifferentiated cells develop into mature adipocytes. Activation of PPARγ promotes the storage of fatty acids in adipose tissue, contributing to the regulation of energy balance in the body [6]. The expression of active PPARγ in


Michael S. Pepper and Melvin A. Ambele (eds.), *Adipogenesis: Methods and Protocols*, Methods in Molecular Biology, vol. 2938, https://doi.org/10.1007/978-1-0716-4607-6_8,

adipocytes or adipose tissue can be detected and measured using the western blot technique. This technique separates protein based on an SDS-PAGE depending on its size. The gel matrix is made from the reaction of acrylamide monomer and bis-acrylamide (N, N′-methylenebisacrylamide) cross-linker that polymerizes to form highly stable horizontal gels. Depending on the ratio of mixed monomer and cross-linker, the gel acts as a sieve through which proteins of different sizes migrate from the negative cathode to the positive anode when voltage is applied [7]. The PPARγ is a 52 kDa protein that can be separated on an ~8% polyacrylamide gel [8]. This chapter describes the western blot protocol for the detection of PPARγ from mature or differentiating adipocytes.

## 2 Materials

### 2.1 Sample Preparation

1. Lysis buffer(s):

   RIPA: 150 mM NaCl, 1% NP-40 or Triton X-100, 0.5% sodium deoxycholate, 0.1% SDS, and 50 mM Tris-HCl, pH 8.0.

   NP-40: 150 mM NaCl, 1% Np-40 or Triton X-100, and 50 mM Tris-HCl, pH 8.0. Tris–HCl: 20 mM Tris–HCl, pH 7.5.

   Chaps: 150 mM KCL, 50 mM HEPES (pH 7.4), and 0.1% CHAPS (*see* **Note 1**).
2. Protease inhibitor cocktail.
3. Phosphate-buffered saline (PBS).

### 2.2 SDS-PAGE

1. Acrylamide/Bis solution: Dissolve 29.2 g of acrylamide monomer, 0.8 g of bis-acrylamide, and a spatula of mixed resin beads in 100 mL of distilled water, to make a 30% acrylamide/bis solution (*see* **Note 2**).
2. Resolving buffer: To make 1.5 M Tris–HCl, pH 8.8 resolving buffer, dissolve 18.15 g of Tris base in 80 mL of distilled water. Change the pH to 8.8 using 6 N HCl. Make up the final volume to 100 mL with distilled water (*see* **Note 3**).
3. Stacking buffer: Prepare 0.5 M Tris–HCl, pH 6.8 stacking buffer by adding 6 g of Tris base in 80 mL of distilled water and adjusting the pH to 6.8 using 6 N HCl. Add more distilled water to make up a final volume to 100 mL (*see* **Note 3**).
4. 2× Laemmli loading buffer: 0.004% bromophenol blue, 10% 2-mercaptoethanol, 20% glycerol, 4% SDS, and 0.125 M Tris–HCl (*see* **Note 4**).
5. One liter of 10× running buffer: Tris–HCl 25 mM (30 g), glycine 200 mM (144 g), and SDS 0.1% (w/v) (10 g).

6. Sodium dodecyl sulfate (SDS): Dissolve 1 g of APS in 10 mL of distilled water to make a 10% solution.
7. Ammonium persulfate (APS): Dissolve 1 g of APS in 10 mL of distilled water to make a 10% solution.
8. N,N,N,N′-Tetramethyl-ethylenediamine (TEMED).

### 2.3 Wet Transfer

1. Filter paper, fiber pads, and nitrocellulose membrane cut to the size of the gel.
2. 10× Tris–glycine: Weigh 30.3 g of Tris base and 144 g of glycine, and add distilled water to a final volume of 1000 mL.
3. Western blot transfer buffer: 1× Tris–glycine—add 100 mL of 10× Tris–glycine, 200 mL of methanol, and 70 mL of distilled water (*see* **Note 5**).
4. Coomassie R250 staining solution: To prepare 0.1% Coomassie Blue R250 (w/w) with 30% methanol and 5% acetic acid, weigh out 1 g of Coomassie R250, and add 300 mL of methanol, 650 mL of distilled water, and 50 mL of acetic acid. Mix with a stir bar on a mixer for 2 h. Filter the solution through a Whatman no. 1 paper, and store at 20 °C.
5. Destain solution: To prepare 30% methanol and 5% acetic acid solution, add 300 mL of methanol and 50 mL of acetic acid to 650 mL of distilled water. Store the solution at 20 °C.
6. Transfer cassettes, module, tank, and power supply.

### 2.4 Immunoblotting and Detection

1. Tris-buffered saline (TBS; 10×): 1.5 M NaCl, 0.1 M Tris–HCl, pH 7.4.
2. TBS containing 0.05% Tween-20 (TBST).
3. Blocking solution. Store it at 4 °C.
4. Primary, for example, anti-PPARγ (rabbit mAb), and secondary antibodies, for example, anti-rabbit IgG.
5. Chemiluminescent ECL substrate.
6. Plastic container.

## 3 Methods

### 3.1 Cell Lysis Using RIPA Buffer

All steps during the protein lysis procedure must be carried out on ice or at 4 °C. At the end of the lysis step, quantification of the extracted protein can be done using BCA Protein Assay Kit.

**Lysis of Monolayer-Cultured Adherent Mammalian Cells**

1. Following ASC adipogenic differentiation and trypsinization (*see* Chap. 7), transfer the cell suspension into a 1.5 mL Eppendorf tube, and centrifuge at 500 × *g* for 5 min.
2. Carefully remove and discard the supernatant.
3. Add chilled/cold PBS onto the pellet, and resuspend the cells; centrifuge at 500 × *g* for 5 min, and then carefully remove and discard the supernatant.
4. Add chilled/cold RIPA lysis buffer (0.5 mL) to the cell pellet, and vortex briefly; then, incubate on ice for 30 min (*see* **Note 6**).
5. Centrifuge the resuspended solution at 14,000 × *g* for 10 min.
6. Carefully aspirate the supernatant, and transfer into a new 1.5 mL Eppendorf tube for further analysis.

**Lysis of Tissue Samples**

1. Rinse the fresh tissue with chilled/cold PBS several times, and grind the tissue into small pieces using a tissue grinder or an appropriate method.
2. For every 1 g of ground tissue sample, add 10 mL of chilled RIPA lysis buffer to it. A smaller volume of buffer can be used if a more concentrated lysate is needed (*see* **Note 6**).
3. Mix the tissue sample for several minutes at high speed until a homogenous consistency is achieved.
4. Leave homogenized tissue sample on ice for 30 min.
5. Centrifuge the tissue sample at approximately 10,000 × *g* for 10 min.
6. Carefully remove the supernatant and transfer into a new tube for further analysis.

### 3.2 SDS-PAGE: Separation of Proteins Based on Size

**Gel Preparation**

1. Using deionized water and ethanol, clean two short glass plates and two spacer plates of the gel casting unit.
2. Place the clean plates on a stable, even surface, and assemble them with the spacers to make two glass cassettes.
3. Slide the glass cassettes into a casting stand, ensuring that the short glass plate is facing the front and that the glass plates are aligned to avoid leakage.
4. Prepare 10 mL of a 10% resolving gel solution by mixing 3.4 mL of acrylamide solution, 2.6 mL of 1.5 M Tris–HCl, pH 8.8, 100 μL of 10% SDS, 100 μL of 10% APS, and 3.8 mL of distilled water. Do *NOT* add TEMED at this point.

### Discontinuous Polyacrylamide Gel Pouring

1. To determine the level to which the resolving gel is poured, insert a comb completely into the assembled glass cassettes, and indicate using a permanent marker on the short glass plate 1 cm below the comb teeth. Remove the comb.
2. Add 100 μL of 10% TEMED to the resolving gel mixture, and immediately pour gently into the tank using a glass or disposable plastic pipette. Overlay the resolving gel solution with water or isopropanol (*see* **Note 7**).
3. Allow the gel to sit for about 45–60 min to allow for polymerization.
4. After polymerization of gel, rinse the gel surface thoroughly with distilled water. The alcohol overlay should not be left on the gel for more than 1 h to avoid dehydrating the top of the gel (*see* **Note 8**).
5. Prepare 10 mL of 5% stacking gel solution by mixing 1.34 mL of 30% acrylamide solution, 2.6 mL of 0.5 M Tris–HCl, pH 6.8, 100 μL of 10% SDS, 100 μL of 10% APS, and 5.86 mL of distilled water.
6. Dry the top of the resolving gel with a filter paper before pouring the stacking gel.
7. Add 100 μL of TEMED to the stacking gel monomer solution and mix.
8. Pour the solution between the glass plates. Continue to pour until the gel reaches the top of the short plate.
9. Place a well comb between the glass plates immediately.
10. Allow the gel to set for about 20–30 min at room temperature.

### Run Gel

1. Remove the gel sandwiches from the casting stand to the clamping frame that has electrodes to create a chamber, making sure that the short glass plates face inward.
2. Fill up the chamber with 1× running buffer such that it washes out the sample wells, and then load the extracted protein samples (~20 μL per well) (*see* **Note 9**).
3. Connect the electrical leads into a power supply, and apply approximately 200 volt power.
4. Run electrophoresis for about 53 min.

### 3.3 Wet/Tank Transfer

**Preparation for Blotting**

1. Cut the nitrocellulose membrane and the filter paper according to the size of the gel. Alternatively, use pre-cut membranes and filter paper.
2. Soak the gel, membrane, filter paper, and fiber pads in the transfer buffer for 15–20 min (*see* **Note 10**).
3. Prepare the gel sandwich by opening and placing the empty cassette in a plastic container, with the black side at the bottom of the container and the clear side against the inner side of the container.
4. Place one presoaked fiber pad on the black side of the cassette.
5. Place three sheets of presoaked filter paper on the fiber pad.
6. Lay the equilibrated gel on the filter paper.
7. Place the presoaked nitrocellulose membrane on top of the gel.
8. Complete the sandwich by placing three more sheets of filter paper on the membrane.
9. Place the last presoaked fiber pad (*see* **Note 11**).
10. Carefully close and lock the cassette firmly, being careful not to distort the sandwich.
11. Insert the cassette in a transfer module, and place the loaded module into a transfer tank.
12. Place a frozen ice pack on one side of the module, and add 1× transfer buffer to the "blotting" mark on the tank.
13. Place a stir bar inside the buffer, and place the tank on top of a magnetic stir bar mixer. Set the speed as fast as possible to keep the ion distribution in the buffer even (*see* **Note 12**).

**Transferring the Protein**

1. Place the lid on; plug the cables into the power supply, and run the transfer for 1 h at 100 V, constant 350 mA.
2. At the end of the run, disconnect the transfer-blot cell, and obtain the blotted membrane by disassembling the sandwich using forceps (*see* **Note 13**).
3. Place the blotted membrane in a 50 mL tube and soak it with TBST.
4. To confirm if the transfer was successful, place the gel in a Coomassie Blue R250 staining solution for 1–4 h on a rocking shaker followed by rinsing with destain solution overnight on rocking shaker (*see* **Note 14**).

### 3.4 Blocking, Immunostaining, and Detection

**Membrane Blocking**

1. Using forceps, transfer the membrane from the 50 mL tube with TBST into a clean 50 mL tube, ensuring that the protein side is facing the inside of the tube.
2. Add 10 mL of blocking buffer to the membrane inside the 50 mL tube, and incubate for 5 min at 4°C with agitation on a roller (*see* **Note 15**).
3. Discard the blocking buffer, and wash the membrane three times for 5 min each using 1× TBST buffer with agitation on a roller.

**Immunostaining**

1. Dilute PPARγ primary antibody of choice to the concentration specified in the manufacturer insert (*see* **Note 16**) in a total volume of 10 mL, and add into the 50 mL tube containing the washed membrane.
2. Incubate for 1 h at room temperature or overnight at 4°C with agitation on a roller.
3. Wash the membrane five times for 5 min each with 1× TBST buffer.
4. Dilute the appropriate secondary antibody (horseradish peroxidase (HRP)-conjugated antibodies, raised against the host species of the corresponding primary antibody) to the concentration specified in the manufacturer insert (*see* **Note 17**) in a total volume of 10 mL, and add into the 50 mL tube containing the washed membrane that has already been stained with the primary antibody.
5. Incubate for 1 h at room temperature or overnight at 4°C with agitation on a roller.
6. Wash the membrane five times for 5 min each with 1× TBST buffer.

**Detection by Chemiluminescent ECL Substrate**

1. Prevent the membrane from drying out by soaking it in the wash buffer in a 50 mL tube while you prepare the substrate mixture.
2. Prepare the substrate kit components by mixing them in a 1:1 ratio (0.1 mL of solution/$cm^2$ of membrane or 7 mL of solution/mini-sized (7 × 8.5 cm) membrane).
3. Discard wash buffer from the membrane, and make sure that the protein side is facing the inside of the tube.

4. Add substrate solution to the blot, and incubate for 5 min on a roller to ensure that the surface of the blot is completely covered with substrate. Avoid air bubbles (*see* **Note 18**).
5. Transfer the membrane from the 50 mL tube using clean blunt forceps, and drain off excess substrate solution.
6. Capture the membrane with a digital imager or by exposure to X-ray film.

## 4 Notes

1. Protein sample preparation for PAGE begins with extracting the sample from its cellular matrix, making it soluble, decontaminating the solution, and standardizing the concentration of the total protein. These steps are necessary for ensuring high-quality starting material for great electrophoresis results and ultimately good western blot data. It is therefore necessary to consider the following factors for an effective extraction of soluble protein samples:
   (a) First, various sample types entail different extraction methods for efficient cell lysis; therefore, choose your method of cell disruption carefully.
   (b) Second, it is important to know the subcellular location of your protein of interest matters, as it will inform the type of method that enriches for that cellular compartment.
   (c) Lastly, different lysis buffers exist based on the detergent composition and can therefore affect the solubilization of different proteins. It is important to choose the appropriate lysis buffer that will yield higher amounts of your target protein.

   For whole cell lysate and membrane-bound protein extraction, RIPA or NP-40 is preferred due to their harsh properties, which make them difficult-to-solubilize proteins. RIPA buffer is recommended for the extraction of nuclear and mitochondrial proteins since it contains SDS detergent, making it well suited for difficult-to-solubilize proteins. Tris–HCl buffer provides optimal conditions for cytoplasmic proteins once an optimal concentration is determined. Other forms of electrophoresis include isoelectric focusing and two-dimensional electrophoresis, which are meant for separating proteins in their native state and thus require uncharged zwitterionic detergents like CHAPS.

2. The acrylamide monomer and the cross-linking agent, bis-acrylamide, are naturally neurotoxins. All the steps must be carried out carefully while wearing powder-free gloves.
3. The stacking gel provides a layer to get all the loaded protein samples lined up to simultaneously enter the separating layer in the resolving gel. The protein samples can move freely in the stacking gel owing to its low percentage of acrylamide, thus facilitating them to reach the resolving gel at the same time. Lowering the pH of the stacking buffer to almost neutral (6.8) helps maintain the uncharged/zwitterionic state of glycine, which, together with the ionated $Cl^-$ from the Tris–HCl buffer, provide constant movement of proteins, allowing them to concentrate and stack into a layer before entering the separating/resolving layer. When they reach the resolving gel, chloride ions and the uncharged glycine lose their neutral state to become negatively charged, which allows them to migrate slowly to the positive anode past the proteins due to the high percentage of acrylamide. The protein samples left behind without a voltage gradient are therefore able to separate.
4. The 2-mercaptoethanol component of the Laemmli loading buffer is a reducing agent that converts a secondary structure of a protein into a primary one. Glycerol helps increase the density of the protein sample to allow it to sink into the wells during loading, while bromophenol blue acts as a tracking dye for monitoring the progress of PAGE gel.
5. To improve heat dissipation, use buffer chilled to 4 °C. You can use ethanol (analytical grade) in place of methanol in all buffer formulations.
6. Pre-chill the required volume of RIPA lysis buffer at 4 °C. Immediately before use, add protease inhibitor and phosphatase inhibitor to the lysis buffer. The chilled RIPA lysis buffer can be added directly to the flask containing cells.
7. The solution should be poured smoothly so that it does not mix with air. For overlaying the poured mixture, do not use butanol or isobutanol.
8. The resolving gel can be stored at room temperature overnight. To store it, add 5 mL of 1:4 dilution of 1.5 M Tris–HCl, pH 8.8 buffer on top of the gel to keep it hydrated.
9. Degradation of proteins in the form of proteolysis, denaturation, and dephosphorylation following cell lysis and solubilization usually occurs almost immediately due to the presence of active enzyme in the sample. To prevent this from happening, a freshly prepared mixture of protease inhibitors should be added to the protein sample while it is kept on ice before while loading the gel or at 4 °C. Several ready-made inhibitor cocktails are available commercially; however, these can be prepared in the lab depending on the needs of individual experiments.

10. Salts from the electrophoresis running buffer can contaminate the transfer buffer by increasing its conductivity and generating more heat during transfer. It is therefore important to pre-equilibrate the gels for 15–20 min in the transfer buffer to facilitate the removal of such contaminants. To prevent further contamination, always wear gloves when handling membranes.
11. Remove any air bubbles that may be trapped in between the sandwich using a glass tube or a roller.
12. To avoid a potential safety hazard and ensure a successful transfer, it is advisable to always place a stir bar inside the transfer buffer and put the tank on a high-speed mixer so that the transfer buffer is constantly stirred during the electrophoretic transfer. This helps to maintain a uniform conductivity and temperature throughout the transfer.
13. At the end of the electrophoretic transfer, rinse the outside cover of the ice pack with water, and return to the freezer for storage.
14. The gel will appear clear or with faint bands upon destaining if transfer was successful.
15. Membrane blocking: Different blocking buffers exist, and the best one will be determined by the type of antibody and membrane used. The amount of time it takes to block a membrane will also affect signal detection. One-hour incubation is recommended; longer durations have the potential to mask epitopes, while shorter durations may lead to high background noise because of nonspecific binding.
16. To determine the optimum antibody concentration, refer to the manufacturer's suggested starting dilution range. A primary antibody binds specifically to a protein of interest that has been immobilized to a membrane.
17. A secondary antibody binds specifically to the isotype and species of a primary antibody to enhance signal and increase detection sensitivity. That is, a goat anti-rabbit secondary is a secondary antibody raised in goats against a primary antibody that was raised in rabbits. Secondary antibodies are conjugated with either enzyme for colorimetric or chemiluminescent detection or with a fluorescent dye for fluorescent detection of the protein of interest.
18. The chemiluminescence chemical reaction is characterized by a chemical reaction where the luminol substrate is oxidized by the horseradish peroxide enzyme that is conjugated to the secondary antibody. This reaction produces a light signal that is captured by a camera or on a film. This light signal is usually weak, which is why luminol must be mixed with enhancers.

## References


1. Mahmood T, Yang PC (2012) Western blot: technique, theory, and trouble shooting. N Am J Med Sci 4:429–434. https://doi.org/10.4103/1947-2714.100998
2. Begum H, Murugesan P, Tangutur AD (2022) Western blotting: a powerful staple in scientific and biomedical research. BioTechniques 73:58–69. https://doi.org/10.2144/btn-2022-0003
3. Gogg S, Nerstedt A, Boren J, Smith U (2019) Human adipose tissue microvascular endothelial cells secrete PPARγ ligands and regulate adipose tissue lipid uptake. JCI Insight 4. https://doi.org/10.1172/jci.insight.125914
4. Ambele MA, Dhanraj P, Giles R, Pepper MS (2020) Adipogenesis: a complex interplay of multiple molecular determinants and pathways. Int J Mol Sci 21. https://doi.org/10.3390/ijms21124283
5. Ma X, Wang D, Zhao W, Xu L (2018) Deciphering the roles of PPARγ in adipocytes via dynamic change of transcription complex. Front Endocrinol (Lausanne) 9:473. https://doi.org/10.3389/fendo.2018.00473
6. Lefterova MI, Haakonsson AK, Lazar MA, Mandrup S (2014) PPARγ and the global map of adipogenesis and beyond. Trends Endocrinol Metab 25:293–302. https://doi.org/10.1016/j.tem.2014.04.001
7. Pillai-Kastoori L, Schutz-Geschwender AR, Harford JA (2020) A systematic approach to quantitative Western blot analysis. Anal Biochem 593:113608. https://doi.org/10.1016/j.ab.2020.113608
8. Gómez D, Guerrero CA (2022) Interaction between proteins of the PPARγ and NFκB immune response pathways and rotavirus non-structural proteins. Acta Virol 66:39–54. https://doi.org/10.4149/av_2022_105

# Chapter 9

# Measurement of Intracellular Reactive Oxygen Species During Adipogenesis

Ladislaus Tapiwa Adam, Melvin A. Ambele, and Michael S. Pepper

## Abstract

Reactive oxygen species (ROS) play an important role in the differentiation of immature stem cells to mature adipocytes in a process known as adipogenesis. Despite decades of study, there is still a gap in our understanding of the exact mechanisms played by ROS in regulating adipogenesis. This chapter describes flow cytometric measurement of endogenous ROS production during adipogenesis in adipose-derived stromal/stem cells (ASCs).

**Key words** Reactive oxygen species, Adipogenesis, MitoSOX™ Red, CellROX® Deep Red reagent, Flow cytometry, Adipose-derived stromal/stem cells (ASCs)

## 1 Introduction

Reactive oxygen species (ROS) are described as unstable oxygen-containing molecules and free radicals, derived exogenously or through endogenous generation in cells as part of various cellular physiological processes [1, 2]. In adipocytes, the main ROS producers are NADPH oxidase 4 (NOX4) and the mitochondria that generate hydrogen peroxide ($H_2O_2$) and superoxide ($O_2^{\bullet -}$), respectively [3–6]. ROS have been implicated in the conversion of stem cells to adipocytes [5–7]. Various methods have been developed to measure ROS levels in cells in vitro. These include direct radical measurements using the electron spin resonance technique; chemiluminescent assays using luminol or lucigenin probes; mitochondria-specific fluorescent probes, e.g., MitoSOX™ Red and MitoTracker Red CM-$H_2$XRos; as well as the cytochrome c reduction, nitro blue tetrazolium, Amplex Red, and dichlorodihydrofluorescein diacetate (DCFH-DA) assays [8, 9]. This protocol describes ROS production measurement during adipogenesis using the CellROX® Deep Red reagent, which detects ROS signals

Michael S. Pepper and Melvin A. Ambele (eds.), *Adipogenesis: Methods and Protocols*, Methods in Molecular Biology, vol. 2938, https://doi.org/10.1007/978-1-0716-4607-6_9,

localized in the cytoplasm, as well as the MitoSOX™ Red mitochondrial superoxide indicator, which detects mitochondrial ROS [10].

## 2 Materials

### 2.1 Cells

Adipose-derived stromal/stem cells at any chosen time point in the adipogenic differentiation process (*see* **Note 1**).

### 2.2 Equipment

1. Laminar air flow cabinet (BSL II).
2. $CO_2$ incubator.
3. Centrifuge.
4. Vacuum aspirator.
5. Flow cytometer.

### 2.3 General Materials and Supplies

1. Pipettes and pipette tips.
2. Centrifuge tubes.
3. Dulbecco's Modified Eagle Medium without pyruvate and without phenol red (*see* **Note 2**).
4. Penicillin/streptomycin (Pen/Strep).
5. Fetal bovine serum (FBS).
6. CellROX® Deep Red reagent (supplied in liquid format as a 2.5 mM stabilized solution in DMSO).
7. MitoSOX™ reagent (supplied in 50 μg powder vials, see Subheading 2.4 for stock solution preparation).
8. Tert-butyl hydroperoxide (TBHP).
9. DAPI stain (supplied in 10 mg powder vials, see Subheading 2.4 for stock solution preparation).
10. Phosphate-buffered saline (PBS); pH 7.4.

### 2.4 Media and Reagent Stock Solutions

1. Complete DMEM (500 mL): Add 50 mL of fetal bovine serum (10% vol/vol) and 10 mL of Pen/Strep (2% vol/vol) to 440 mL of DMEM. Carefully swirl the bottle around a few times to ensure proper mixing, and keep refrigerated between 4 and 8 °C.
2. MitoSOX™: Prepare 5 mM of MitoSOX™ reagent stock solution. Dissolve the contents (50 μg) of one vial of MitoSOX™ mitochondrial superoxide indicator in 13 μL DMSO.
3. DAPI: Prepare 5 mg/mL of DAPI stock solution. Dissolve the contents of one vial (10 mg) in 2 mL of deionized water. For long-term storage, the stock solution can be aliquoted and stored at ≤ −20 °C. Prepare a 10 μg/mL of DAPI working

solution in staining buffer [100 mM Tris Buffer (pH 7.4), 150 mM NaCl, 1 mM $CaCl_2$, 0.5 mM $MgCl_2$] by pipetting 2 μL DAPI stock solution to 1 mL staining buffer.

## 3 Methods

### 3.1 CellROX® Deep Red Assay

1. At the time points chosen to measure ROS in differentiated cells, discard the cell culture or adipogenic differentiation medium (*see* **Note 3**).
2. Add 4 mL of sterile PBS to the cells.
3. Carefully swirl the flask around to ensure the PBS washes around the entire cell surface; then, discard the PBS. Repeat this PBS wash step twice.
4. Add 4 mL of 0.25% trypsin-EDTA to cells inside the T80 culture flask.
5. Incubate flask at 37 °C and 5% $CO_2$ for about 7 min.
6. Check under the microscope to make sure all the cells have detached from the bottom of the flask. If majority of cells have not detached, prolong the incubation time by a further 5 min and observe again under the microscope to make sure cells have dislodged from the bottom of the flask into suspension.
7. Add 4 mL of complete DMEM medium to the flasks to neutralize the enzymatic activity of 0.25% trypsin-EDTA on the cells.
8. Transfer the cell suspension into a sterile 15 mL Eppendorf tube.
9. Centrifuge the cell suspension at 300 × *g* for 5 min to pellet cells, and discard the supernatant.
10. Add 4 mL of complete DMEM to cell pellet, and carefully resuspend the cells by pipetting gently up and down (*see* **Note 4**).
11. Pipette 1 mL of cell suspension into a flow cytometry tube (*see* **Note 4**).
12. Set up a tert-butyl hydroperoxide (TBHP) positive control tube as follows:

    Pipette 1 mL of ASC cell suspension (undifferentiation control cells) into a flow cytometry tube, and add 100 μM of TBHP; then, incubate for 30 min at 37 °C (*see* **Note 5**). Thereafter, this TBHP positive control tube should follow the same procedural steps as the test cell suspension (adipogenic differentiated cells) as described below.
13. Add 1 μL of CellROX® Deep Red reagent to all cell suspensions to make a final concentration of 5 μM (*see* **Note 6**).

14. Add 0.5 μL of DAPI working solution to cell suspensions to make a final concentration of 5 ng/mL (*see* **Note 7**).
15. Incubate in the dark at 37 °C for 30 min.
16. Centrifuge the cell suspension at 300 × *g* for 5 min to pellet the cells, and discard the supernatant.
17. Add 1 mL of PBS to the cell pellet and repeat **step 16** twice.
18. Resuspend in 1 mL of complete DMEM (or PBS supplemented with 10% of FBS), and analyze immediately using a flow cytometer (*see* **Note 8**).

### 3.2 MitoSOX™ Red Assay

1. At the time points chosen to measure ROS in the adipogenic differentiated cells, discard the cell culture or adipogenic differentiation medium (*see* **Note 3**).
2. Add 4 mL of sterile PBS to cells.
3. Carefully swirl the flask around to ensure the PBS washes around the entire cell surface, and then discard the PBS. Repeat this PBS wash step twice.
4. Add 4 mL of 0.25% trypsin-EDTA to cells inside the T80 culture flask.
5. Incubate the flask at 37 °C and 5% $CO_2$ for about 7 min.
6. Check under the microscope to make sure cells have detached from the bottom of the flask. If the majority of cells have not detached, prolong incubation time by a further 5 min, and observe again under the microscope to make sure cells have dislodged from the bottom of the flask into suspension.
7. Add 4 mL of complete DMEM to the flasks to neutralize the enzymatic activity of the 0.25% trypsin-EDTA on the cells.
8. Transfer the cell suspension into a sterile 15 mL Eppendorf tube.
9. Centrifuge the cell suspension at 300 × *g* for 5 min to pellet cells, and discard the supernatant.
10. Add 4 mL of complete DMEM to the cell pellet, and carefully resuspend the cells by pipetting gently up and down (*see* **Note 4**).
11. Pipette 1 mL of cell suspension into a flow cytometry tube (*see* **Note 4**).
12. Add 1 μL MitoSOX™ reagent to cell suspension to make a final concentration of 5 μM (*see* **Note 6**).
13. Add 0.5 μL DAPI working solution to cell suspension to make a final concentration of 5 ng/mL (*see* **Note 7**).
14. Incubate in the dark at 37 °C for 30 min.

15. Centrifuge the cell suspension at 300 × *g* for 5 min to pellet cells, and discard the supernatant.
16. Add 1 mL of PBS to cell pellet and repeat **step 5** twice.
17. Resuspend in 1 mL of complete DMEM (or PBS supplemented with 10% of FBS), and analyze immediately using a flow cytometer (*see* **Note 8**).

## 4 Notes

1. Adipogenesis experiments described in this method were performed in T80 flasks. However, other flask sizes and plates can be used. In other experiments in our laboratory, 6-well plates and 12-well plates have been used for experiments where high cell numbers were not required. There were no significant differences in adipogenic differentiation observed between cells cultured in 6-well and 12-well plates when compared to those differentiated in T80 flasks.
2. Use DMEM without pyruvate and phenol because pyruvate is a ROS scavenger that may influence the results if present in culture medium [11, 12]. Phenol, on the other hand, interferes with florescence and flow cytometry measurements [13].
3. Set up a negative control ASC plate composed of non-adipogenic induced, untreated ASCs to detect any changes in either cell viability or intracellular ROS levels during adipogenesis. Negative control ASCs follow the same procedural steps as the test cells.
4. Care should be taken when handling delicate cells such as adipocytes. It is advised to minimize additional washing steps to prevent release of intracellular lipid droplets by differentiated adipocytes. Use pipette tips with wide bore or disposable Pasteur pipettes for cell suspension transfers.
5. Tert-butyl hydroperoxide (tBHP) induces ROS production in the cells and thus acts as a positive control for the assay.
6. In stem cells and adipocytes, the major ROS sources are NOX4 and mitochondrial-derived ROS [3, 4]. As such, this method outlines ROS measurements during adipogenesis using the CellROX® Deep Red reagent, which detects ROS signals localized in the cytoplasm, and MitoSOX™ Red is a mitochondrial superoxide indicator which detects mitochondrial ROS.
7. DAPI is a DNA binding dye that only penetrates cells with compromised membranes and is therefore an indicator of cell death. Once the dye enters the cell, it binds to DNA and fluoresces. The fluorescent cells represent dead cells and can therefore be gated out during flow cytometric analysis.

**Table 1**
**The excitation and emission spectrums, lasers, and detectors used for all fluorochrome and/or dyes used in the experiments**

| Reagent | Excitation laser | Emission wavelength | Filter | Detection channel |
|---|---|---|---|---|
| MitoSOX™ | Blue: 488 nM | 580 nM | 575/30 | FL2 |
| CellROX® | Red: 638 nM | 665 nM | 620/20 | FL6 |
| DAPI | Violet: 405 nM | 461 nM | 450/40 | FL9 |

8. A Gallios flow cytometer was used in our experiments. Instrument start-up was performed, and Flow Check Pro™ fluorospheres were used to verify laser alignment and instrument performance. Acquisition protocols on the instrument were set to acquire 5000 events, with a second stop criterion of not exceeding an acquisition time of 5 min for each sample. Following data acquisition on the Gallios flow cytometer, data analysis was done using the Kaluza analysis software version 2.0. Table 1 shows the excitation lasers and detection (emission) channels for the different fluorochromes.

To ensure that data analysis was done only on viable cells with intact membranes, the following gating strategy was implemented using Kaluza analysis software. Gating strategies were set using non-adipogenic induced, untreated ASCs, which served as the negative control. These settings were then applied to the rest of the conditions throughout the differentiation period to detect any changes in either cell viability or intracellular ROS levels. First-level gating was done to identify viable ASCs, and this was done by creating a side scatter (SS) Log vs DAPI FL9 density plot (Fig. 1a). A region was then drawn on the DAPI dim population, which represented viable ASCs. The DAPI bright cells represented dead cells and were gated out as shown in Fig. 1a. Thereafter, a forward scatter (FS) vs side scatter (SS) Log density plot was created, and this was gated on the viable cells (Fig. 1b). This was to exclude debris as well as any remaining dead cells. Dead cells and debris tend to have lower FS levels and are usually located at the bottom left corner of the FS/SS density plot. A region was drawn on the intact cells leaving out the debris, as shown in Fig. 1b, and these cells were identified as the ASCs.

For intracellular ROS assay setup and gating strategy, in the case of CellROX® Deep Red assay, a SS Log vs CellROX® FL6 density plot on ASCs was created to detect total intracellular ROS levels (Fig. 2a). An SS Log vs MitoSOX™ FL2 plot on ASCs was created to detect mitochondrial ROS levels (Fig. 2b). Mean fluorescence intensity (MFI) was the parameter used to assess intracellular ROS levels. MFI represents the quantity of a parameter per

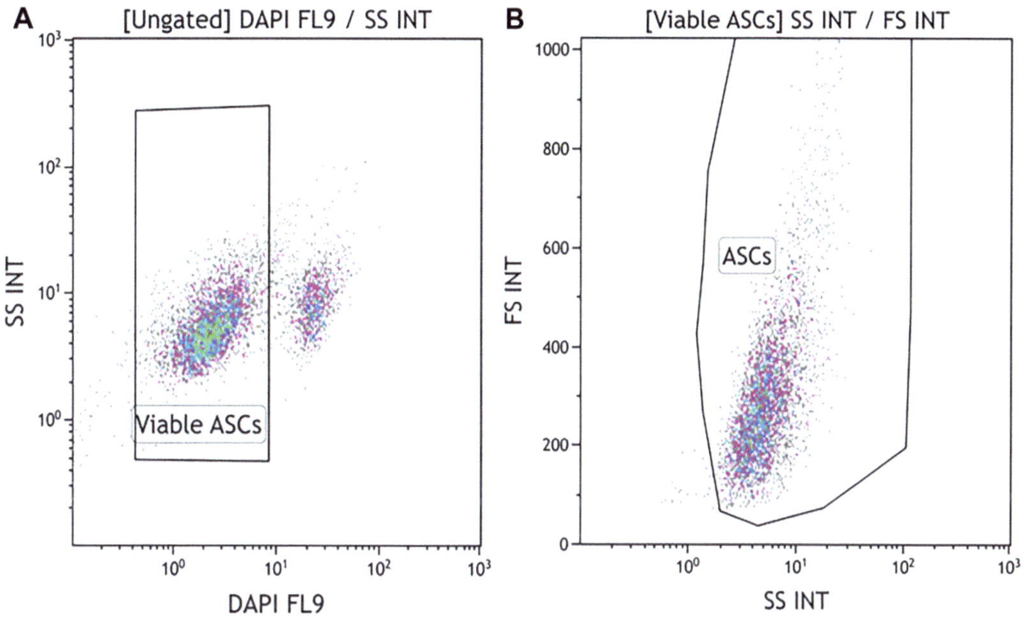


**Fig. 1** Gating strategy for viable and intact ASCs. Non-adipogenic induced, untreated ASCs were used to set the gating controls. Only viable cells were used for data analysis; dead cells and debris were removed from analysis. DAPI bright cells represented dead cells and were excluded from analysis (**a**). Debris and the remaining dead cells were excluded using the FS vs SS density plot (**b**)

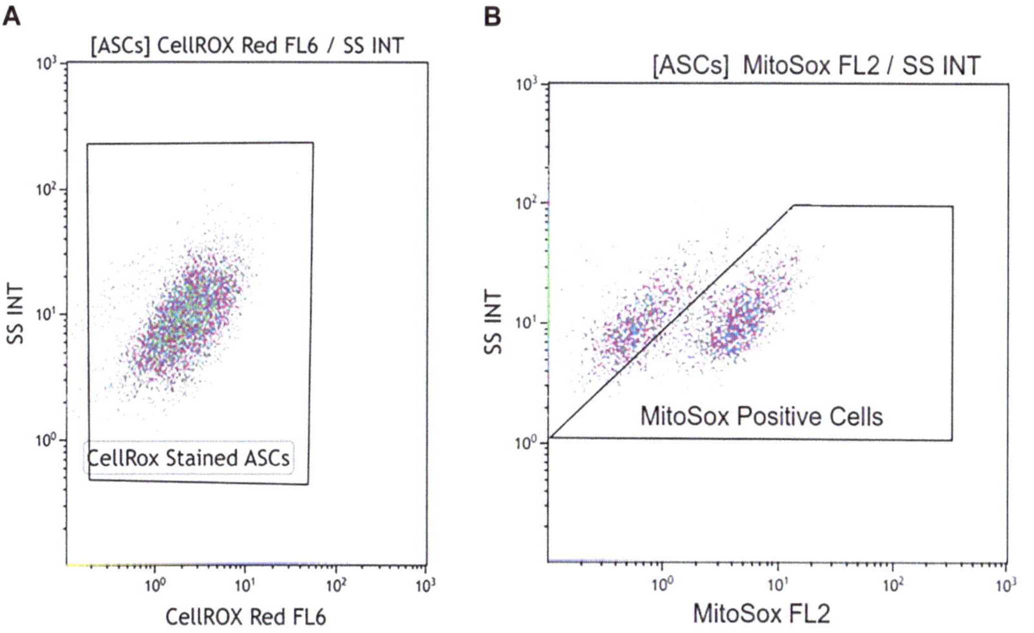


**Fig. 2** Gating strategy to detect intracellular ROS levels in differentiating ASCs. Total intracellular cytoplasmic ROS levels were measured from the MFI of the cells in the CellROX Red FL6 region (**a**). Mitochondrial ROS levels were represented by MitoSOX positive cells in the MitoSOX FL2 region (**b**)

event, in other words the fluorescence intensity per cell, and expressed as relative fluorescent units. All cells stained positive with the CellROX® Deep Red reagent; thus, a region was drawn around all cells, as shown in Fig. 2a. Interestingly, we observed a MitoSOX Red negative and a MitoSOX Red positive population. Thus, for MitoSOX Red, we reported the MFI of the cells that stained positive for MitoSOX Red. For the MFI, a region was drawn around the proportion of cells that stained positively with MitoSOX™ Red reagent as shown in Fig. 2b.

## References

1. Prasad S, Gupta SC, Tyagi AK (2017) Reactive oxygen species (ROS) and cancer: role of antioxidative nutraceuticals. Cancer Lett 387:95–105. https://doi.org/10.1016/J.CANLET.2016.03.042
2. Galadari S, Rahman A, Pallichankandy S, Thayyullathil F (2017) Reactive oxygen species and cancer paradox: to promote or to suppress? Free Radic Biol Med 104:144–164. https://doi.org/10.1016/J.FREERADBIOMED.2017.01.004
3. Liu Y, Fiskum G, Schubert D (2002) Generation of reactive oxygen species by the mitochondrial electron transport chain. J Neurochem 80:780–787
4. Dikalov S (2011) Cross talk between mitochondria and NADPH oxidases. Free Radic Biol Med 51:1289–1301. https://doi.org/10.1016/j.freeradbiomed.2011.06.033
5. Furukawa S, Fujita T, Shimabukuro M et al (2004) Increased oxidative stress in obesity and its impact on metabolic syndrome. J Clin Invest 114:1752–1761. https://doi.org/10.1172/JCI200421625.1752
6. Higuchi M, Dusting GJ, Peshavariya H et al (2013) Differentiation of human adipose-derived stem cells into fat involves reactive oxygen species and forkhead box O1 mediated upregulation of antioxidant enzymes. Stem Cells Dev 22:878–888. https://doi.org/10.1089/scd.2012.0306
7. Kanda Y, Hinata T, Won S, Watanabe Y (2011) Reactive oxygen species mediate adipocyte differentiation in mesenchymal stem cells. Life Sci 89:250–258. https://doi.org/10.1016/j.lfs.2011.06.007
8. Eruslanov E, Kusmartsev S (2010) Identification of ROS using oxidized DCFDA and flow-cytometry. Methods Mol Biol 594:57–72. https://doi.org/10.1007/978-1-60761-411-1
9. Wiederschain GYA (2010) Molecular probes handbook, a guide to fluorescent probes and labeling technologies, 11th edn. Molecular Probes
10. Life Technologies Corporation (2012) CellROX ® oxidative stress reagents, pp 1–6
11. Long LH, Halliwell B (2009) Artefacts in cell culture: pyruvate as a scavenger of hydrogen peroxide generated by ascorbate or epigallocatechin gallate in cell culture media. Biochem Biophys Res Commun 388:700–704. https://doi.org/10.1016/j.bbrc.2009.08.069
12. Ramos-Ibeas P, Barandalla M, Colleoni S, Lazzari G (2017) Pyruvate antioxidant roles in human fibroblasts and embryonic stem cells. Mol Cell Biochem 429:137–150. https://doi.org/10.1007/s11010-017-2942-z
13. Wu D, Yotnda P (2011) Production and detection of Reactive Oxygen Species (ROS) in cancers. J Vis Exp e3357. https://doi.org/10.3791/3357

# Chapter 10

# Oxygen Consumption and Extracellular Acidification Rate in Adipogenic Differentiated Human Mesenchymal Stromal/Stem Cells

**Miguel Angel Olmedo-Suárez, Edgar Sánchez-Ramírez, Ximena del Toro-Rios, Lilia G. Noriega, and Lorena Aguilar-Arnal**

## Abstract

Human mesenchymal stem/stromal cells (hMSCs) constitute a primary cell source in adipogenesis, playing a pivotal role in the generation of new adipocytes. This process is accompanied by substantial metabolic shifts in hMSCs, notably characterized by a transition from glycolytic to oxidative metabolism. Monitoring metabolic alterations during adipogenic differentiation can be achieved through the assessment of extracellular flux parameters, such as the oxygen consumption rate (OCR) and extracellular acidification rate (ECAR). In this study, we provide a comprehensive protocol for differentiating hMSCs into the adipogenic lineage, with an emphasis on tracking differentiation stages through extracellular flux measurements. We determined the cellular metabolic status throughout the adipogenic differentiation by assessing OCR and ECAR to gauge mitochondrial respiration and glycolytic activity, respectively, using a Seahorse XFe96 extracellular flux analyzer.

**Key words** Human mesenchymal stem/stromal cells, Adipogenesis, Extracellular flux, Glycolysis, Oxidative phosphorylation, Extracellular acidification, Oxygen consumption, Mitochondrial respiration, Seahorse extracellular flux analyzer

## 1 Introduction

During adipogenesis, new adipocytes develop and accumulate in various locations within the body, including subcutaneous fat deposits [1]. Human mesenchymal stem/stromal cells (hMSCs), also known as multipotent stromal cells, play a pivotal role in adipocyte generation [2]. Notably, both hMSCs residing within

Authors Miguel Angel Olmedo-Suárez and Edgar Sánchez-Ramírez have equally contributed to this chapter.

Michael S. Pepper and Melvin A. Ambele (eds.), *Adipogenesis: Methods and Protocols*, Methods in Molecular Biology, vol. 2938, https://doi.org/10.1007/978-1-0716-4607-6_10,

the adipose tissue and those derived from bone marrow have been implicated in adipogenesis in adult animals [2, 3]. hMSCs are nonhematopoietic progenitor cells found in adult tissues, exhibiting significant proliferative potential in an undifferentiated state and the capacity to differentiate into various mesenchymal lineages when exposed to appropriate stimuli [4]. Furthermore, hMSCs are under consideration for therapeutic applications in a range of human diseases, including neurodegenerative disorders, cardiovascular conditions, and diabetes [5].

Like many other types of stem cells, hMSCs primarily rely on glycolysis for energy production in their undifferentiated state, subsequently transitioning to oxidative phosphorylation (OXPHOS) in mitochondria during differentiation [6, 7]. The development of adipocytes involves two primary steps: (1) commitment of hMSCs to preadipocytes and (2) differentiation of preadipocytes into mature adipocytes [8]. Throughout this adipogenic process, tight regulation occurs at transcriptional, epigenomic, and metabolic levels, involving the production of reactive oxygen species (ROS) [9–12]. As these changes unfold, mitochondrial biogenesis and cellular oxygen consumption increase compared to undifferentiated control cells, while lactate production decreases [13].

For the detection of metabolic alterations in cells, the measurement of the cellular oxygen consumption rate (OCR) and extracellular acidification rate (ECAR) serves as valuable extracellular flux parameters to estimate mitochondrial respiration and glycolysis, respectively [14, 15]. The Seahorse extracellular flux analyzer (XFe96) continuously tracks changes in oxygen concentration and proton flux in the cell culture medium over time [14]. The OCR parameter has been effectively utilized to assess the enhancement in respiratory capacity of hMSCs in comparison to undifferentiated hMSCs during adipogenic commitment. Furthermore, ECAR measurements reflect that undifferentiated hMSCs exhibit a glycolytic phenotype. Therefore, these extracellular flux parameters have proven to be valuable for monitoring metabolic shifts during adipogenic differentiation [12].

Here, we present a protocol for evaluating the metabolic profiles of differentiating hMSCs into adipocytes by measuring extracellular flux parameters (OCR and ECAR). Adipogenic differentiation is induced in actively growing hMSCs (70–80% confluency) [12, 16]. Subsequently, the metabolic status during the adipogenic process is assessed using the Seahorse XFe96 extracellular flux analyzer. This equipment allows for the simultaneous measurement of both OCR and ECAR in live cells, presented in a 96-well plate format. This protocol outlines the optimal parameters for extracellular flux analysis specifically tailored to hMSCs.

## 2 Materials

### *2.1 Equipment*

1. Cell culture incubator set to 37 °C and 5% $CO_2$.
2. Non-$CO_2$, 37 °C incubator with humidified environment (i.e., a tray of water inside).
3. Clean centrifuge for 15 mL tubes containing cells.
4. Water bath set to 37 °C.
5. Laminar flow hood.
6. Neubauer chamber or automated cell counter. Here, we use the LUNA-II™ system (Logos Biosystems) and the cell imaging multimode reader Cytation 1 (BioTek).
7. Inverted microscope connected to a camera.
8. Seahorse XFe96 extracellular flux analyzer (Agilent) (Figs. 1 and 2a).

### *2.2 Reagents and Materials for Cell Culture and Maintenance*

1. Human bone marrow-derived mesenchymal stem/stromal cells (BM-hMSCs). These cells can be obtained from healthy donors with ethics considerations and informed consent provided. Alternatively, a commercial cell line of BM-hMSCs

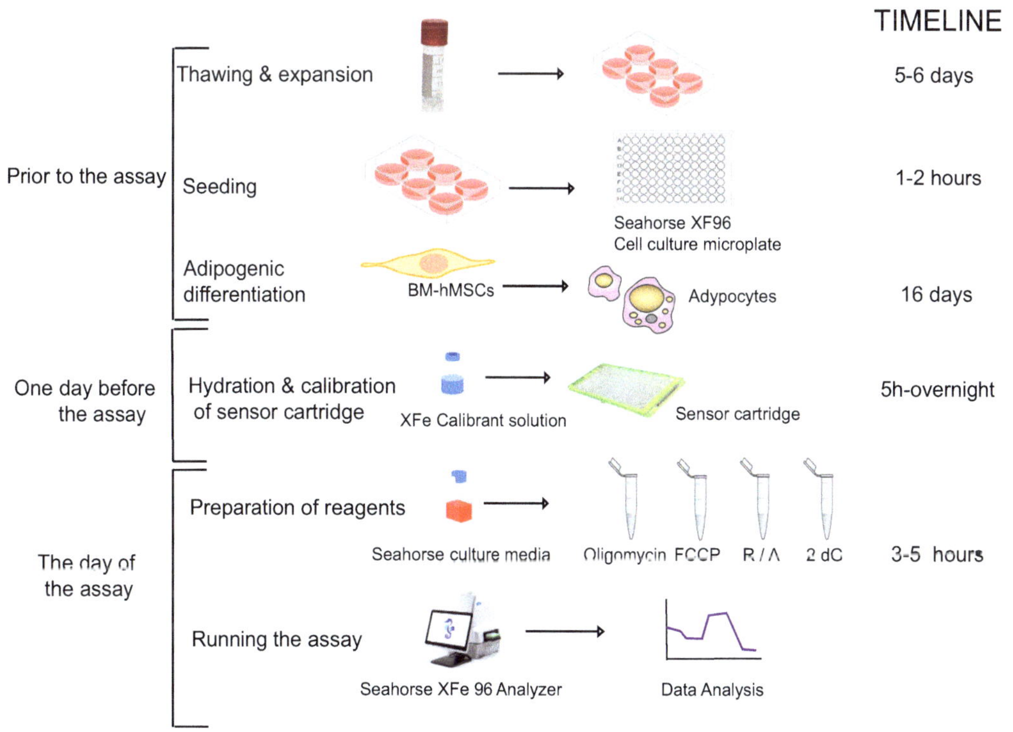


**Fig. 1** Overview of the entire process. The workflow consists of preparing the cells for the analyses, preparing the equipment, and assessing the OCR and ECAR using the Seahorse extracellular flux analyzer

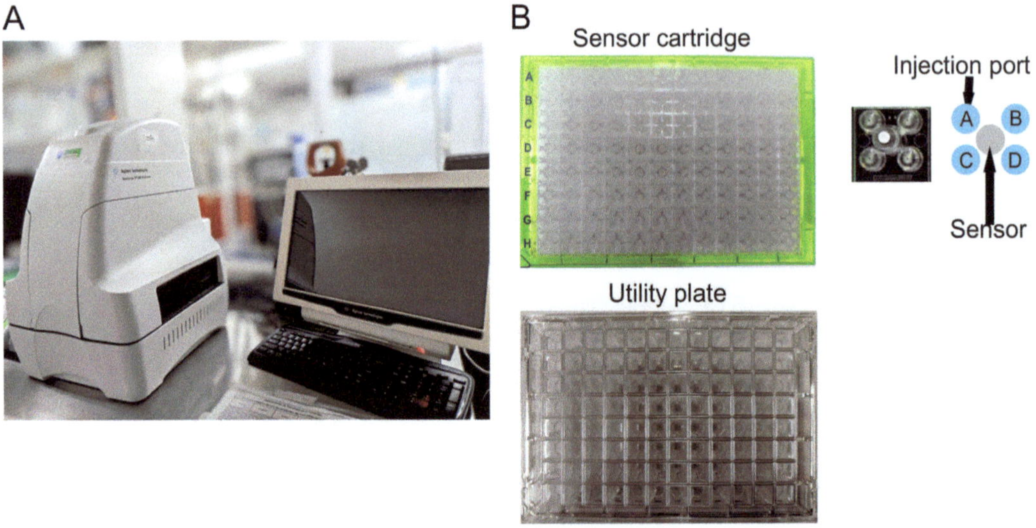


**Fig. 2** Equipment used for the extracellular flux analysis assay. (**a**) Extracellular flux analyzer Seahorse XFe96 (**b**) Sensor cartridges and utility plate

can be obtained from ATCC (Cat. No. PCS-500-012) (*see* **Note 1**).

2. hMSC maintenance medium: Dulbecco's Modified Eagle Medium (DMEM), low glucose.
3. Fetal bovine serum.
4. L-Glutamine solution 200 mM.
5. Penicillin–streptomycin solution 100×.
6. 100 mM non-TC treated culture dish (p100).
7. 0.4% trypan blue solution.
8. Dulbecco's Phosphate Buffered Saline (DPBS).
9. Adipogenic differentiation medium: StemPro® Adipogenesis Differentiation Kit. Thaw the supplement provided in the kit in a 37 °C water bath, and add it to the basal medium (10% final concentration) and antibiotic solution (1%). The supplemented adipogenic differentiation medium should be stored at 2–8 °C in the dark for up to a month.
10. Trypsin solution: 2.5 mL of 1× DPBS was added to a 7.5 mL aliquot of 0.25% trypsin-EDTA 0.25% in phenol red to have a final concentration of 0.18%. This dilution makes the cell detachment process less aggressive.

### 2.3 Reagents and Materials for Extracellular Flux Analysis

1. Fibronectin.
2. Seahorse XF assay medium: The Seahorse XF DMEM medium is DMEM-based and must be supplemented with 1 mM pyruvate, 2 mM glutamine, and 10 mM D-glucose, pH 7.4.
3. Oligomycin A: Prepare a 2.5 mM stock solution by dissolving 5 mg of oligomycin in 2.53 mL of dimethylsulfoxide (DMSO). Prepare 20 μL aliquots of the solution, and store them at −20 °C.
4. Carbonyl cyanide-p-trifluoromethoxyphenylhydrazone (FCCP): Prepare a 39.3 mM solution by dissolving 10 mg FCCP in 1 mL of DMSO. Then, dilute the desired amount to a 2.5 mM stock solution. Prepare 20 μL aliquots of the solution, and store them at −20 °C.
5. Rotenone: Prepare a 181 mM solution by dissolving 1 g of rotenone in 14 mL of DMSO. Then, dilute the desired amount to a 2.5 mM stock solution. Prepare 20 μL aliquots of the solution, and store them at −20 °C.
6. Antimycin A: Prepare a 45.6 mM solution by dissolving 25 mg of antimycin in 1 mL of DMSO. Then, dilute the desired amount to a 2.5 mM stock solution. Prepare 20 μL aliquots of the solution, and store them at −20 °C.
7. 2-Deoxy-D-glucose: On the day of the assay, prepare a 500 mM stock solution by dissolving 250 mg of 2-deoxy-D-glucose in 3 mL of Seahorse XF assay medium.
8. Hoechst 33342: Prepare a 17.8 mM stock solution by dissolving 10 mg of Hoechst 33342 in 1 mL of DMSO. Prepare 20 μL aliquots, and store them at −20 °C.
9. From each stock solution, prepare working solutions load into the injection ports on sensor cartridges.

**Table 1**
**Preparation of working solutions of respiration modulators**

| Port and compounds | Stock solution conc. | Stock solution quantity | Media volume (μL) | 10× (Port) | Volume added to port (μL) | Final conc. Per well |
|---|---|---|---|---|---|---|
| Port A Oligomycin | 2.5 mM | 24 μL | 3000 | 20 μM | 20 | 2.0 μM |
| Port B FCCP | 2.5 mM | 6 μL | 3000 | 5 μM | 22 | 0.5 μM |
| Port C Rot/AA | 2.5 mM | 6/6 μL | 3000 | 5/5 μM | 25 | 0.5/0.5 μM |
| Port D 2DG | N/A (powder) | 0.250 g | 3000 | 500 mM | 27 | 50 mM |

10. Prepare 3 mL volume of working solutions for each respiratory modulator in the Seahorse XF assay medium (*see* **Note 2**). The optimized concentrations of working solutions for this assay consist of oligomycin 2 μM, FCCP 0.5 μM, Rot/AA 0.5 μM each, and 2-deoxy-D-glucose 50 mM (Table 1) (*see* **Note 3**).
11. Seahorse XFe96/XF Pro FluxPak: Includes 18 XFe96/XF Pro sensor cartridges,18 XFe96/XF Pro Cell Culture Microplates, and 1 bottle of Seahorse XF Calibrant Solution 500 mL.

## 3 Methods

The complete experimental procedure is shown in Fig. 1 with all the procedures performed at room temperature under sterile or clean conditions unless otherwise specified. The procedure comprises three stages.

1. Cell thawing and expansion.
2. Preparation of the sensor cartridge 1 day before the assay.
3. Preparation of the working solutions, measurements, and analyses to determine OCR and ECAR on the day of the assay.

### 3.1 Cell Culture and Adipogenic Differentiation in hMSCs

1. Add 7.5 mL of DMEM low glucose to four 100 mM cell culture plates, and put them in the $CO_2$ incubator at 37 °C for 1 h.
2. Prepare a sterile and pre-labeled 15 mL conical tube with 8 mL of DMEM low glucose, and allow it to equilibrate to 37 °C in a water bath.
3. Retrieve a cryovial with the hMSCs, containing approximately 500,000–1 million cells, from the liquid nitrogen tank, and proceed immediately to thaw them in a 37 °C water bath by carefully submerging the cryovial, ensuring that the lid does not come into contact with the water's surface.
4. Gently agitate the vial from side to side until a small ice pellet forms at the bottom.
5. Immediately, wipe down the cryovial with 70% alcohol, and then remove excess water with a sterile dry towel.
6. Open the cryovial in the hood and collect the cells using a 1000 μL pipette.
7. Gently transfer them into the 15 mL tube from **step 1**.
8. Centrifuge at 1300 × *g* for 5 min at room temperature, and discard the supernatant.
9. Resuspend the cell pellet in 10 mL of fresh medium to obtain a cellular suspension of approximately 50,000 cells/mL.
10. Add 2.5 mL of cellular suspension (approximately 125,000 cells) to each of the four prepared Petri dishes from **step 1**.

11. Gently swirl the dishes to evenly distribute the cells, and place them in the incubator at 37 °C with 5% $CO_2$.
12. Change the medium every 3 days until cells reach 70–80% confluence (*see* **Note 4**).

### 3.2 Seed Cells into the Agilent Seahorse XF96/XF Pro Cell Culture Microplates

1. Prepare the Agilent Seahorse XF96/XF Pro Cell Culture Microplate by adding 20 μL of a 10 μg/mL solution of human fibronectin.
2. Incubate at 37 °C inside the cell culture incubator for 2 hours.
3. Aspirate the fibronectin, and leave the plates inside the hood for 20 min at room temperature. After that, plates are ready for seeding.
4. Take the hMSCs out from the incubator, and wash twice with 5 mL of DPBS inside the hood.
5. Add 3 mL of trypsin solution, and incubate for 4 minutes at 37 °C inside the incubator (*see* **Note 5**).
6. Add 3 mL of DMEM low glucose supplemented with 10% of FBS to inactivate the trypsin.
7. Using a 10 mL pipette, collect the cells and deposit them into a 15 mL conical tube.
8. Centrifuge for 5 minutes at 1300 × *g* at room temperature.
9. Discard the supernatant and resuspend the cells in 1 mL of fresh medium.
10. Count live cells using 0.4% trypan blue and an automated cell counter or a Neubauer chamber.
11. Calculate the volume needed to seed 10,000 cells, and add it to each well of the Agilent Seahorse XF96/XF Pro Cell Culture Microplate (*see* **Note 6**). It is recommended to seed 6–10 wells per experimental condition for technical replicates. We suggest avoiding seeding cells in the perimeter wells of the microplate, as these have been observed to introduce significant variation. Thus, add only medium to the perimeter wells. Seed a number of plates equal to the planned days for adipogenesis analysis. For example, five plates are required to investigate days 0 (hMSCs), 4, 8, 12, and 16 after adipogenic induction (*see* **Note 7**).
12. Add 100 μL/well of hMSC maintenance medium to the plate designated for day 0.
13. Add 100 μL/well of adipogenic differentiation medium to the remaining plates.
14. Incubate the plates inside the incubator for 2 days to facilitate cell recovery.
15. Then, proceed with the OCR and ECAR measurements of the day 0 plate using the extracellular flux analyzer Seahorse XFe96.

16. For the other plates, replace the medium every 4 days. Note that the procedure of measuring OCR and ECAR begins the day before the assay with the preparation of the XFe96/XF Pro sensor cartridge.

### 3.3 Extracellular Flux Analyzer Seahorse XFe96 and Configuration of the Assay

For the extracellular flux analysis assay (*see* **Note 8**), there are preparations to be done the day before the assay and on the day of the assay.

*Day before the assay—sensor cartridge hydration.*

1. Hydrate a sensor cartridge plate: Separate the sensor cartridge (green) from the utility plate (transparent), and apply 100 μL/well of the Seahorse XF Calibrant Solution to the utility plate.
2. Carefully immerse the sensor cartridge back into the utility plate to allow hydration.
3. Place inside the non-$CO_2$ incubator at 37 °C overnight, together with a tray of water to prevent evaporation.

*Day of assay—running the extracellular flux analysis.*

1. Switch on the Seahorse XFe96 extracellular flux analyzer and the controller; then, open the "Wave" software to indicate the analyzer to reach 37 °C.
2. Prepare enough Seahorse XF assay medium, and warm it to 37 °C in a water bath (calculate 500 mL/well).
3. Carefully wash the cells cultured in the XF Cell Culture Microplate by replacing the differentiation medium with XF assay medium (add 200 μL/well and remove).
4. Add 180 μL/well of XF assay medium, and incubate the plate at 37 °C for 30 minutes into the non-$CO_2$ incubator, including the perimetral wells which will serve as background measurements.
5. Prepare and charge the working solutions in the ports of the cartridge: In port A, add 20 μL of 10× (20 μM) oligomycin for a final concentration of 2 μM in the well. In port B, add 22 μL of 10× (5 μM) FCCP for a final concentration of 0.5 μM in the well. In port C, add 25 μL of a 10× mixture (5 μM each) of rotenone/antimycin for a final concentration of 0.5 μM each. Finally, in port D, add 27 μL of the 2-deoxy-D-glucose 500 mM solution with Hoechst 33342 for a final concentration of 50 mM and 2 μM, respectively, in the well (*see* **Note 9**).
6. Program the assay in the wave software: Enter your experiment settings by selecting XF Cell Mito Stress Test from the Templates window. Then, fill the Plate map tab with your experimental setup and indicate the parameters in the Protocol tab, also adding injection for port D. Thus, the protocol consists of five sets of measurements: baseline, oligomycin (port A), FCCP

(port B), rotenone + antimycin A (port C), and 2-deoxy-D-glucose (port D). Each set is composed of three measurements cycles as follows: 3 min mix, 0 min wait, and 3 min measure. Indicate the program to Start Run, and save your assay in a dedicated location.

7. The first part of the assay is the calibration procedure. Insert the sensor cartridge in the tray, and let the calibration process take place for approximately 20 min.
8. After the calibration procedure, remove the utility plate, and insert the XF96 Cell Culture Microplate on the tray with the cell culture.
9. Then, start the run.
10. When the run is complete, count the number of nuclei per well using the Cytation 1 platform and the Gen5 software.
11. Normalize the data with regard to the number of nuclei by using the normalization tab in the wave software.
12. Generate your OCR data report (*see* **Note 10**).

## 4 Notes

1. Plasticware and liquids used for cell culture and adipogenic differentiation must be sterile. Store all reagents at 4 °C, and allow them to reach room temperature before their use with cells. Avoid heating reagents and media. For reagents stored at −20 °C, prevent repeated freeze–thaw cycles by aliquoting them into smaller volumes. Prepare all solutions using ultrapure water (generated by purifying deionized water) and analytical-grade reagents. When working with cells, ensure that you wear gloves, and protective eyewear is recommended for added safety.
2. Use the compounds on the same day that they are reconstituted. The remaining compound solutions should not be reused or repeatedly frozen.
3. The optimal final compound concentration for achieving maximal effect is cell line dependent and may be affected by assay medium types. Use these recommendations for hMSCs.
4. Cells at passage 6 or lower yield the best differentiation rates.
5. If the trypsin is fresh, 4 min may suffice to detach the cells. However, if the trypsin has undergone repeated freeze–thaw cycles or if it is over a month old, an extended incubation of 5 min may be required.
6. The accuracy in cell counting is important for lowering the variability of the assay. Cells should be plated uniformly and in a

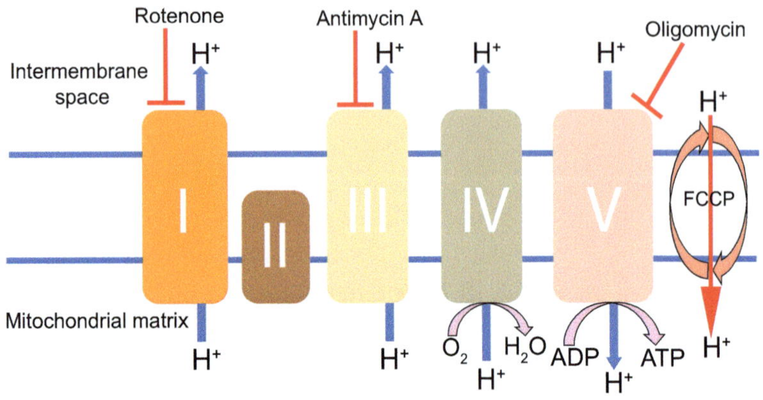


**Fig. 3** Scheme of action of respiration modulators. Oligomycin inhibits mitochondrial ATP synthase; FCCP uncouples the mitochondrial proton gradient from ATP synthase function; rotenone inhibits complex I, and antimycin inhibits complex III of the electron transport chain. 2-Deoxy-D-glucose is finally added and inhibits the hexokinase activity (not shown here)

monolayer configuration. Cell clusters may cause poor cell adhesion and inaccurate measurements.

7. Using the StemPro adipogenic differentiation kit, adipogenic differentiation from hMSCs is achieved in 16 days. During this process, sequential and specific fluctuations in transcriptional patterns occur in concert with metabolic rewiring. Consequently, cells progressively accumulate lipids, which can be visualized with Oil Red O staining if desired (Fig. 5).

8. For extracellular flux analysis assay, the equipment includes the Seahorse XFe96 extracellular flux analyzer with a controller and registration computer, a non-$CO_2$ incubator, and a cell imaging multimode reader (Fig. 2a). The extracellular flux measurements (OCR and ECAR) are optimized for a 96 well-plate format and the use of built-in injection ports on the XFe96/XF Pro sensor cartridges (Fig. 2b). The equipment sequentially adds the modulators of cellular respiration: oligomycin, FCCP, rotenone–antimycin, and 2-deoxy-D-glucose, to detect key parameters of mitochondrial function (Fig. 3). Briefly, oligomycin inhibits mitochondrial ATP synthase. The resulting drop in OCR is attributed to the ATP-linked oxygen consumption, and the concomitant rise in ECAR is due to the compensation of glycolysis for the loss of mitochondrial ATP production. FCCP uncouples the mitochondrial proton gradient from ATP synthase function, hereby driving maximal oxygen consumption. Rotenone inhibits complex I, and antimycin inhibits complex III of the electron transport chain; hence, both hinder mitochondrial respirations. Therefore, residual oxygen consumption is regarded as non-mitochondrial respiration. Finally,

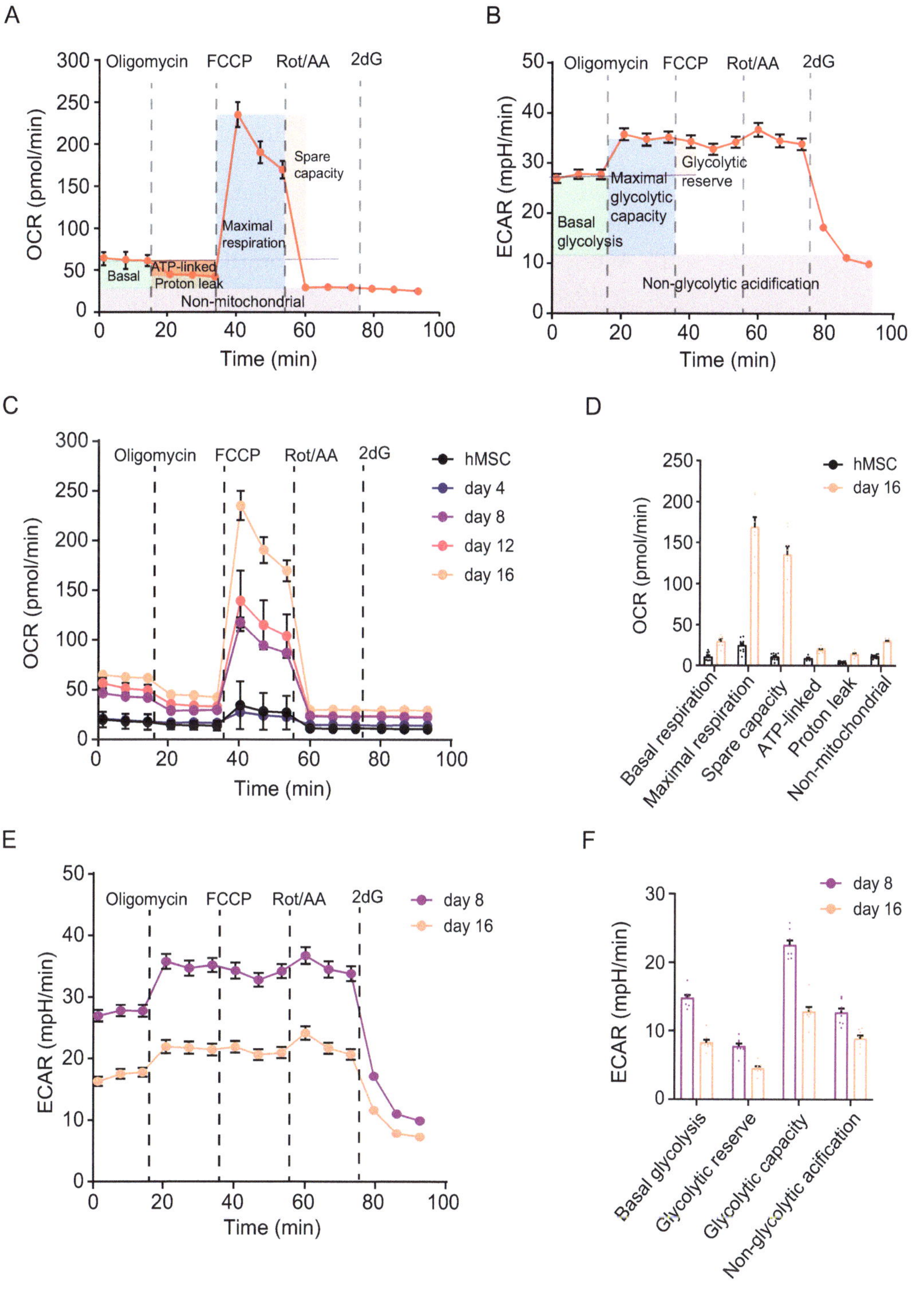


**Fig. 4** Examples of OCR and ECAR measurements. (**a**) The fundamental parameters of mitochondrial bioenergetics: basal respiration, ATP turnover, proton leak, maximal respiration, and spare respiratory capacity can be calculated from the OCR data normalized to the number of cells. (**b**) The glycolytic parameters can be estimated from the ECAR measurements. Basal glycolysis is determined by subtracting the average

by adding 2-deoxy-D-glucose, an inhibitor of hexokinase activity, we can estimate basal glycolysis, glycolytic capacity, and glycolytic reserve. The residual ECAR is considered as non-glycolytic acidification (Fig. 4a, b).

9. We recommend adding 3 μL of Hoechst 33342 to the 3 mL 2-deoxy-D-glucose solution to be injected together to the wells. This will allow to stain the cellular nuclei for normalization of the data to the number of cells.

10. When the assay is finished and normalized, the Seahorse XF Mito Stress Test Report Generator automatically calculates the Seahorse XF Cell Mito Stress Test parameters from the Seahorse software data that has been exported to Excel. The Seahorse XF Stress Test Report Generator provides a convenient, customizable, one-page assay summary. Additionally, other software including GraphPad are convenient to plot the data and determine statistical significance. The OCR and ECAR

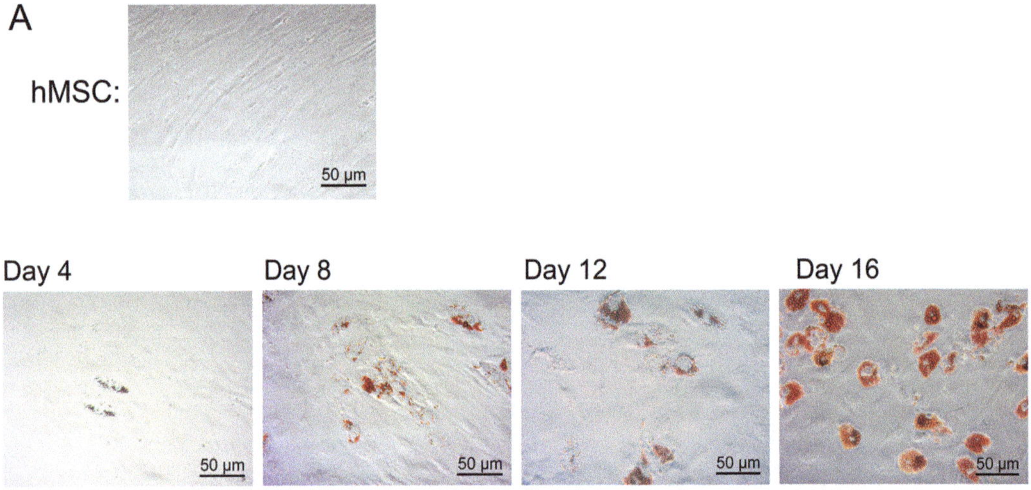


**Fig. 5** ORO staining of hMSCs during adipogenic differentiation. (**a**) The staining was performed before adipogenic induction (upper panel, hMSC), and at days 4, 8, 12, and 16 after adipogenic induction

**Fig. 4** (continued) ECAR after 2-deoxyglucose injection from the average basal ECAR; glycolytic reserve is determined by subtracting the average basal ECAR from the average ECAR after oligomycin injection, and glycolytic capacity is determined by subtracting the average ECAR after 2-deoxyglucose injection from the average ECAR after oligomycin injection. (**c**) Examples of real-time OCR measurements from hMSCs before and after adipogenic induction at the indicated days. (**d**) Determination of the parameters of mitochondrial bioenergetics from hMSCs before and after adipogenic differentiation. (**e**) Examples of real-time ECAR measurements at day 8 and at terminal (day 16) adipogenic differentiation from hMSCs. F) Determination of glycolytic flux from ECAR measurements at days 8 and 16 (terminal) after adipogenic induction from hMSCs. Data was normalized to number of cells normalized to cell number are plotted against time to show the metabolic response to each compound (Fig. 4). During adipogenesis, increased OCR can be seen as hMSCs develop through the adipogenic process. It is expected to find substantial differences in OCR between undifferentiated hMSC and terminally differentiated adipocytes [13]. Parallel measurement of the ECAR as an indication of the glycolytic rate can confirm that hMS cells rely mostly on aerobic glycolysis as an energy source.

## Acknowledgements

We acknowledge all the members of LA-A and LGN labs for helpful scientific discussions and advice. We acknowledge MSc Marcia Bustamante Zepeda at the Instituto de Investigaciones Biomedicas—UNAM for technical advice. This work was funded by DGAPA-PAPIIT IN204325 from Universidad Nacional Autónoma de México (UNAM), the Chan Zuckerberg Initiative Grant 2023-331942 (5022) GB-1597645, and the National Council of Science and Technology (CONACyT) FORDECYT-PRONACES/15758/2020, to LA-A. MAOS was supported by a postdoctoral fellowship from DGAPA-UNAM.

### References

1. Sarjeant K, Stephens JM (2012) Adipogenesis. Cold Spring Harb Perspect Biol 4:a008417. https://doi.org/10.1101/cshperspect.a008417
2. Matsushita K, Dzau VJ (2017) Mesenchymal stem cells in obesity: insights for translational applications. Lab Investig 97:1158–1166. https://doi.org/10.1038/labinvest.2017.42
3. Lee RH, Kim B, Choi I, Kim H, Choi HS, Suh K, Bae YC, Jung JS (2004) Characterization and expression analysis of mesenchymal stem cells from human bone marrow and adipose tissue. Cell Physiol Biochem 14:311–324. https://doi.org/10.1159/000080341
4. Ding DC, Shyu WC, Lin SZ (2011) Mesenchymal stem cells. Cell Transplant 20:5–14. https://doi.org/10.3727/096368910x
5. Lv M, Zhang S, Jiang B, Cao S, Dong Y, Cao L, Guo S (2021) Adipose-derived stem cells regulate metabolic homeostasis and delay aging by promoting mitophagy. FASEB J 35:e21709. https://doi.org/10.1096/fj.202100332R
6. Varum S, Rodrigues AS, Moura MB, Momcilovic O, Easley CAT, Ramalho-Santos J, Van Houten B, Schatten G (2011) Energy metabolism in human pluripotent stem cells and their differentiated counterparts. PLoS One 6:e20914. https://doi.org/10.1371/journal.pone.0020914
7. Shum LC, White NS, Mills BN, Bentley KL, Eliseev RA (2016) Energy metabolism in mesenchymal stem cells during osteogenic differentiation. Stem Cells Dev 25:114–122. https://doi.org/10.1089/scd.2015.0193
8. Li S-N, Wu J-F (2020) TGF-β/SMAD signaling regulation of mesenchymal stem cells in adipocyte commitment. Stem Cell Res Ther 11:41. https://doi.org/10.1186/s13287-020-1552-y
9. Ghaben AL, Scherer PE (2019) Adipogenesis and metabolic health. Nat Rev Mol Cell Biol 20:242–258. https://doi.org/10.1038/s41580-018-0093-z
10. Shyh-Chang N, Daley GQ, Cantley LC (2013) Stem cell metabolism in tissue development and aging. Development 140:2535–2547. https://doi.org/10.1242/dev.091777
11. Tormos KV, Anso E, Hamanaka RB, Eisenbart J, Joseph J, Kalyanaraman B, Chandel NS (2011) Mitochondrial complex III ROS regulate adipocyte differentiation. Cell Metab 14:537–544. https://doi.org/10.1016/j.cmet.2011.08.007

12. Sánchez-Ramírez E, Ung TPL, Alarcón Del Carmen A, del Toro-Ríos X, Fajardo-Orduña GR, Noriega LG, Cortés-Morales VA, Tovar AR, Montesinos JJ, Orozco-Solís R, Stringari C, Aguilar-Arnal L (2022) Coordinated metabolic transitions and gene expression by NAD+ during adipogenesis. J Cell Biol 221. https://doi.org/10.1083/jcb.202111137
13. Zhang Y, Marsboom G, Toth PT, Rehman J (2013) Mitochondrial respiration regulates adipogenic differentiation of human mesenchymal stem cells. PLoS One 8:e77077. https://doi.org/10.1371/journal.pone.0077077
14. Wu M, Neilson A, Swift AL, Moran R, Tamagnine J, Parslow D, Armistead S, Lemire K, Orrell J, Teich J, Chomicz S, Ferrick DA (2007) Multiparameter metabolic analysis reveals a close link between attenuated mitochondrial bioenergetic function and enhanced glycolysis dependency in human tumor cells. Am J Physiol Cell Physiol 292:C125–C136. https://doi.org/10.1152/ajpcell.00247.2006
15. Plitzko B, Loesgen S (2018) Measurement of oxygen consumption rate (OCR) and Extracellular Acidification Rate (ECAR) in culture cells for assessment of the energy metabolism. Bio Protoc 8:e2850. https://doi.org/10.21769/BioProtoc.2850
16. Aguilar-Arnal L, Ranjit S, Stringari C, Orozco-Solis R, Gratton E, Sassone-Corsi P (2016) Spatial dynamics of SIRT1 and the subnuclear distribution of NADH species. Proc Natl Acad Sci USA 113:12715–12720. https://doi.org/10.1073/pnas.1609227113

# Chapter 11

# In Vitro Expansion of Human Adipose-Derived Stem Cells (ASCs)

**Ladislaus Tapiwa Adam, Melvin A. Ambele, and Michael S. Pepper**

## Abstract

Adipose-derived stromal/stem cells (ASCs) have raised a great deal of interest in research and regenerative medicine with potential applications in the treatment of several diseases. ASCs are often required in large numbers for use in research and clinical applications. Standardization of isolation methods, expansion, and characterization will ensure quality of the cells as well as safety in their use. This protocol describes the expansion and characterization of ASCs and highlights ASC viability assessment following expansion.

**Key words** Adipose-derived stromal/stem cells, Characterization, Cell expansion, Flow cytometry, Cell culture

## 1 Introduction

Adipose-derived stromal/stem cells (ASCs) have generated great interest both in research and their potential clinical applications in several areas [1]. ASCs can be harvested with relative ease from adipose tissue and can be expanded in vitro using simple techniques. Their ease of isolation and expansion has led to numerous protocols being described in literature making standardization of techniques difficult [2]. In vitro expansion of ASCs is most commonly performed using the monolayer cell culture technique in standard medium (DMEM or α-MEM) supplemented with 10% fetal bovine serum or 10% human platelet lysate (hPL) [3, 4]. Procedures involved in the harvesting and processing of ASCs have been reported to alter physiological characteristics such as the growth rate and tri-lineage differentiation of the isolated stem cells [3, 5]. Thus, to confirm that cells are representative of ACSs, guidelines of the International Federation for Adipose Therapeutics and Science (IFATS) together with the International Society for Cellular Therapy (ISCT) are commonly adopted. Based on these criteria, the cells should be plastic adherent and positive for cell

Michael S. Pepper and Melvin A. Ambele (eds.), *Adipogenesis: Methods and Protocols*, Methods in Molecular Biology, vol. 2938, https://doi.org/10.1007/978-1-0716-4607-6_11,

surface markers CD13, CD29, CD44, CD73, CD90, and CD105; CD36 and CD34 are unstable positive markers present at variable levels. The cells should also be negative for the markers CD31, CD45, and CD235a [6–8]. This protocol describes the procedures used in the expansion, characterization, and viability assessment of expanded ASCs.

## 2 Materials

Human adipose-derived stromal/stem cells (ASCs) freshly isolated or cryopreserved can be used. ASCs can be isolated from either lipoaspirates or solid fat tissue samples.

### 2.1 Equipment

1. Laminar air flow cabinet (BSL II).
2. $CO_2$ incubator.
3. Centrifuge.
4. Vacuum aspirator.
5. Inverted microscope.
6. Flow cytometer.

### 2.2 General Materials and Supplies

1. Tissue culture plates and flasks.
2. Pipettes and pipette tips.
3. Centrifuge tubes.
4. Flow cytometry tubes.
5. Dulbecco's Modified Eagle Medium.
6. Penicillin/streptomycin (Pen/Strep).
7. Fetal bovine serum (FBS).
8. Trypsin-EDTA (0.25%).
9. 7-Aminoactinomycin D.
10. Phosphate-buffered saline (PBS); pH ~ 7.4.
11. Monoclonal antibody solutions CD34, CD45, CD73, CD90, CD36, and CD44.
12. Complete DMEM medium (500 mL): From a 500 mL medium bottle, remove 60 mL, and transfer to a 50 ml centrifuge tube (this aliquot can be stored for future use). Add 50 mL fetal bovine serum (10% vol/vol) and 10 mL Pen/Strep (2% vol/vol) to the remaining 440 mL medium. Gently invert the bottle a few times to ensure proper mixing, and keep refrigerated at 2–8 °C.

## 3 Methods

### 3.1 Expansion of ASCs (in T80 Flasks)

1. Add 8 mL of complete DMEM medium into a sterile T80 culture flask.
2. Transfer 1 mL of resuspended freshly isolated cells into T80 flasks to a seeding density of 5000 cells/cm$^2$ (*see* **Note 1**).
3. Mix evenly, and maintain ASCs at normal culture conditions in an incubator at 37 °C and 5% $CO_2$ (*see* **Note 2**).
4. After 24 h, wash cells by aspirating the medium and replacing it with 8 mL of complete DMEM medium. Change medium after every 3–4 days (*see* **Note 3**).
5. At 80–90% confluency, discard cell culture medium.
6. Add 4 mL of sterile PBS to cells.
7. Carefully swirl the flask around to ensure the PBS washes around the entire cell surface, and then discard the PBS.
8. Repeat the PBS wash **steps 6** and **7** three times to make sure the complete DMEM medium is completely washed off the cells.
9. Add 4 mL of 0.25% trypsin-EDTA to cells inside the T80 culture flask.
10. Incubate flask at 37 °C and 5% $CO_2$ for about 7 min.
11. Check under the microscope if more than 90% of the cells have detached from the bottom of the flask. If majority of cells have not detached, prolong the incubation time by 5 more minutes, and observe again under the microscope to make sure cells have dislodged from the bottom of the flask.
12. Add 4 mL of complete DMEM medium to the flasks to neutralize the enzymatic action of the 0.25% trypsin-EDTA.
13. Transfer the cell suspension into a sterile 15 mL Eppendorf tube.
14. Centrifuge the cell suspension at 300×*g* for 5 min to pellet cells, and discard the supernatant.
15. Add 4 mL of complete DMEM medium to cell pellet, and carefully resuspend the cells by pipetting gently up and down.
16. Repeat **steps 14** and **15** twice, leaving behind a clean cell pellet free of 0.25% trypsin-EDTA.
17. Resuspend the clean cell pellet in 1–2 mL of complete medium (*see* **Note 4**).
18. Perform cell counts using an appropriate method, and reseed cells at a density of 5000 cells/cm$^2$ in T80 flasks.

19. Repeat the **steps 5–18** until the required number of cells is reached for the planned experiment or assay in question (*see* **Note 5**).
20. Any remaining cells can be cryopreserved in DMEM supplemented with 10% DMSO, and store in liquid nitrogen for future use.

### 3.2 Flow Cytometric Characterization of ASCs

1. Pipette 100 μL of cell suspension to a flow cytometry tube.
2. Add 5 μL of antibody solutions of CD34, CD45, CD73, CD90, CD36, and CD44 (*see* **Note 6**).
3. Incubate for 20 min in the dark at room temperature.
4. Add 700 μL of PBS to the flow cytometry tube followed by analyses on a flow cytometer.
5. Set up a second flow cytometry tube containing 100 μL of cell suspension without any antibodies to serve as an unstained negative control (*see* **Note 7**).

### 3.3 ASC Viability Assessment During Expansion

1. Pipette 100 μL of the cell suspension to a flow cytometry tube.
2. Add 5 μL of 7-aminoactinomycin D (7-AAD).
3. Incubate in the dark for 15 min at 37 °C.
4. Add 700 μL of PBS.
5. Run on flow cytometer (*see* **Note 8**).

## 4 Notes

1. As an alternative, the following two adjustments can be adopted to ensure cells are evenly spread on the flask surface:
   (a) Transfer 8 mL of cell suspension (seeding density adjusted to 5000 cells/cm$^2$) in complete DMEM medium to flask.
   (b) First transfer 4 mL complete DMEM medium into a flask, and spread the medium evenly on the flask surface, and then add 4 mL cell suspension (seeding density adjusted to 5000 cells/cm$^2$) in complete DMEM medium to flask to make it a total of 8 mL.
2. Gently move the plate back and forth and then side to side. Leave it to stand on a flat surface (away from vibrations/motion) for 30 min before final incubation. This technique has helped ensure seeded ASCs are evenly spread on flask surfaces.
3. Washing is done to remove any floating debris or dead cells. Cultures have been shown to be unaffected with medium changes of up to once every 7 days. Regular checks of cultures for contamination and yellowing of medium are recommended to ensure cells are well maintained in culture.

4. Volume will depend on cell pellet size; increase medium volume as appropriate. Pellets of cells pooled from between 2 and 10 T80 flasks, 2–5 mL medium volume for reconstitution is recommended.
5. Whenever previously cultured cells are trypsinized and reseeded, the passage number increases by one, e.g., Passage 0 (P0) becomes P1. Take note that with increasing passage number, ASCs undergo morphological transformations accompanied by progressive changes in phenotype. Based on experiments performed in our laboratory, adipogenic differentiation of human ASCs was best at passages below P7; an increase in cell passage numbers of between P10 and P14 showed a significant decrease in adipogenic differentiation capacity [9].
6. To ensure that the cells used adhere to the ASCs' recommended immunophenotype, use a six-color antibody immunophenotype panel as recommended per the criteria set out by the International Federation for Adipose Therapeutics and Science (IFATS) and International Society of Cellular Therapy (ISCT) [6, 8, 10].
7. The negative control tube serves as a baseline onto which positive detection limits are set for the stained sample.
8. Various factors, including cell culture conditions and sample preparation, may compromise sample viability. It is thus important to monitor cell viability during sample analysis.

## Acknowledgements

This work was supported by the South African Medical Research Council (Extramural Unit for Stem Cell Research and Therapy) and the University of Pretoria via the Institute for Cellular and Molecular Medicine.

### References

1. Helmy MA, Mohamed AF, Rasheed HM, Fayad AI (2020) A protocol for primary isolation and culture of adipose-derived stem cells and their phenotypic profile. Alex J Med 56: 42–50. https://doi.org/10.1080/20905068 2020.1750863
2. Si Z, Wang X, Sun C et al (2019) Adipose-derived stem cells: sources, potency, and implications for regenerative therapies. Biomed Pharmacother 114:108765. https://doi.org/10.1016/J.BIOPHA.2019.108765
3. Palumbo P, Lombardi F, Siragusa G et al (2018) Methods of isolation, characterization and expansion of human adipose-derived stem cells (ASCs): an overview. Int J Mol Sci 19: 1897
4. Czapla J, Matuszczak S, Kulik K et al (2019) The effect of culture media on large-scale expansion and characteristic of adipose tissue-derived mesenchymal stromal cells. Stem Cell Res Ther 10:1–11. https://doi.org/10.1186/S13287-019-1331-9/FIGURES/6

5. Riis S, Zachar V, Boucher S et al (2015) Critical steps in the isolation and expansion of adipose-derived stem cells for translational therapy. Expert Rev Mol Med 17:e11. https://doi.org/10.1017/ERM.2015.10
6. Baer PC (2014) Adipose-derived mesenchymal stromal/stem cells: an update on their phenotype in vivo and in vitro. World J Stem Cells 6:256–265. https://doi.org/10.4252/wjsc.v6.i3.256
7. Bourin P, Bunnell BA, Casteilla L et al (2013) Stromal cells from the adipose tissue-derived stromal vascular fraction and culture expanded adipose tissue-derived stromal/stem cells: a joint statement of the International Federation for Adipose Therapeutics (IFATS) and Science and the International Society for Cellular Therapy (ISCT). Cytotherapy 15:641–648. https://doi.org/10.1016/j.jcyt.2013.02.006. Stromal
8. Oberbauer E, Steffenhagen C, Wurzer C et al (2015) Enzymatic and non-enzymatic isolation systems for adipose tissue-derived cells: current state of the art. Cell Regen 4(4):7. https://doi.org/10.1186/S13619-015-0020-0
9. Safwani WKZW, Makpol S, Sathapan S, Chua K (2014) Impact of adipogenic differentiation on stemness and osteogenic gene expression in extensive culture of human adipose-derived stem cells. Arch Med Sci 10:597–606. https://doi.org/10.5114/aoms.2014.43753
10. Oberbauer E, Steffenhagen C, Wurzer C et al (2015) Enzymatic and non-enzymatic isolation systems for adipose tissue-derived cells: current state of the art. Cell Regen 4. https://doi.org/10.1186/S13619-015-0020-0

# Chapter 12

# siRNA Silencing of Adipogenic Gene in ASCs

**Pontsho Moela**

## Abstract

The most common technique used in silencing gene expression adopts a naturally occurring cellular process called RNA interference (RNAi), which uses a double-stranded RNA molecule to silence homologous endogenous genes by degrading their cognate mRNA transcripts. The presence of long double-stranded RNA molecules triggers this process, which ensues by first shortening the lengthy transcripts enzymatically followed by their incorporation into the RISC complex thus allowing it to find and degrade complementary mRNA sequences. In an in vitro setting, short interfering oligonucleotides are commercially synthesized and commonly transfected into mammalian cells through lipofection. This current chapter illustrates the silencing of PPARγ gene using RNAi in adherent mammalian cells.

**Key words** RNA interference, siRNA, Lipofection, Adipogenesis, PPARγ

## 1 Introduction

Experimental tools that allow specific silencing of target genes are powerful technologies that hold promise for scientific research. The most common technique used in this context adopts a naturally occurring cellular process called RNA interference (RNAi), which uses a double-stranded RNA molecule to silence homologous endogenous genes by degrading their cognate mRNA transcripts [1]. RNAi is a posttranscriptional event that plays a role in silencing transposons and regulating gene expression, particularly during embryonic development. It is triggered by the presence of long double-stranded RNA (dsRNA), which get converted into short double-stranded oligonucleotides, also called as small interfering RNAs (siRNAs), which lead to gene silencing in a sequence-specific manner [2]. During the RNAi pathway, the long double-stranded RNA molecules are cleaved by the endoribonuclease called Dicer, which is a member of the RNase III family of enzymes [3], into 19–23 nucleotide siRNAs with 5′ phosphorylated ends and 2-nucleotide unpaired and unphosphorylated 3′ ends [4]. Each double-stranded siRNA is made up of a guide strand and a

Michael S. Pepper and Melvin A. Ambele (eds.), *Adipogenesis: Methods and Protocols*, Methods in Molecular Biology, vol. 2938, https://doi.org/10.1007/978-1-0716-4607-6_12,

passenger strand that get unwound by another enzyme called endonuclease Argonaute 2 (Ago 2) [5]. Once unwound, the guide strand is incorporated into a multicomponent nuclease called the RNA interference specificity complex (RISC) to confer target specificity to the enzyme, while the passenger strand gets discarded. The target-specific RISC enzyme is now able to find complementary mRNA sequences, leading to their endonucleolytic cleavage [6].

When applied **in vitro**, the RNAi process is triggered by the introduction of synthetic siRNA oligonucleotides since long dsRNA could lead to the activation of the immune system in mammalian cells. This bypasses the stage of cleavage by Dicer. The process of introducing external genetic material into a mammalian cell is called transfection, and different modes of transfection exist, such as viral transfection, electroporation microinjection, and lipofection [7]. Lipofection involves the use of liposome as vectors for delivering genetic material into a mammalian cell through fusion with the lipid bilayer of the cell [7]. PPARγ is a nuclear receptor protein that plays a key role in the regulation of adipogenesis by promoting the differentiation of stem cells into adipocytes and promoting fatty acid storage in adipose tissue [8]. Previously, a study found that PPARγ silencing suppressed adipogenesis and stimulates a higher level of matrix mineralization in human adipose-derived mesenchymal stem cells (ASCs) [9]. In this chapter, a comprehensive procedure of PPARγ gene silencing by RNAi is illustrated using the lipofection method of transfection in mammalian cells.

## 2 Materials

1. siRNA oligonucleotide targeted to the gene of interest: PPARγ (Hs01 00218390 and Hs01 00218391).
2. Transfection reagent (liposome).
3. Reduced serum growth medium.
4. Microcentrifuge tubes.
5. Mammalian adherent cells.
6. Six-well plate.
7. cDNA.
8. Forward (3′ CGTGGATCTCTCCGTAAT 5′) and reverse (3′ TGGATCTGTTCTTGTGAATG 5′) primers of PPARγ.
9. SYBR Green master mix.
10. Thermal cycler.

## 3 Methods

### 3.1 Resuspension of siRNA for Use with Transfection Reagent

We recommend that you prepare 10 μM siRNA stock solutions.

1. Briefly centrifuge the vial containing the lyophilized siRNA to ensure that it settles at the bottom of the tube.
2. Resuspend the siRNA in nuclease-free water at a final concentration of 10 μM (50 μL for 0.5 nmol siRNA).
3. To avoid significant degradation of siRNA oligonucleotides, aliquot the solution into two or more vials to limit the number of freeze–thaw cycles of the oligos.
4. Store the oligos at −80 °C in a freezer until use (*see* **Note 1**).

### 3.2 Preparation of Transfection reagent–siRNA Complexes

We recommend using 10 nM final siRNA concentration as a starting point.

1. Dilute 3.75–7.5 μL of lipofectamine reagent in 125 μL of reduced serum medium (*see* **Note 2**).
2. Dilute 2–8 μL of 10 μM siRNA with 125 μL of reduced serum medium (*see* **Note 2**).
3. Mix the diluted siRNA with diluted lipofectamine in a 1:1 ratio, and incubate for 5 min at RT.

### 3.3 Transfection reagent–siRNA Delivery into Cells

1. Seed cells at preferred seeding density, and allow cells to reach 60–80% confluency at the time of transfection (*see* **Note 3**).
2. Wash adherent cells twice with 1 mL of PBS.
3. Add 250 μL/well of the siRNA–transfection reagent complex solution directly onto adherent cells, and mix gently to overlay the mixture over the washed cells.
4. Incubate the cells for 2–3 days in a 37 °C incubator, and then analyze cells (*see* **Note 4**),

### 3.4 Gene Expression Analysis Post-transfection Using the $2^{-\Delta\Delta C_T}$ (Livak) RT-qPCR Method

1. Types of samples to prepare:
   (a) Test samples (transfected): one with the target gene, PPARγ, and another with reference gene, e.g., GAPDH.
   (b) Calibrator samples (non-transfected): one with target the gene, PPARγ, and another reference gene, e.g., GAPDH.
2. Prepare a 10 μL of reaction mixture per sample, in triplicates, containing:
   (a) 0.5 μL of sample buffer.
   (b) 0.5 μL of SYBR Green master mix.
   (c) 0.5 μL of forward primer and 0.5 μL reverse primers specific to gene of interest.

   (d) 2 μL of cDNA template (1000 μg/mL) (*see* **Note 5**).
   (e) 6.5 μL of nuclease-free $dH_2O$.
3. Run RT-qPCR under the following cycling conditions:
   (a) 95 °C for 2 min to activate polymerase.
   (b) 95 °C for 15 s to denature the double-stranded cDNA template and 60 °C for 1 min for primer annealing. Set the thermal cycler to repeat this over 40 cycles (*see* **Note 6**).
   (c) Set the following conditions for constructing a melting curve: 95 °C for 15 s, 60 °C for 1 min, and 95 °C for 15 s (*see* **Note 7**).

### 3.5 The $2^{-\Delta\Delta C_T}$ (Livak) Method

To use the Livak method for relative gene expression calculation, first establish that both target and reference genes are amplified with efficiencies near 100% and within 5% of each other. This can then be followed by determining the relative difference in expression level of the target gene in different samples by following the steps below:

1. Normalize the Cq of the target gene to that of the reference (ref) gene for both the test sample and the calibrator sample:

$$\Delta Cq_{(\text{test})} = Cq_{(\text{target,test})} - Cq_{(\text{ref,test})}$$

$$\Delta Cq_{(\text{calibrator})} = Cq_{(\text{target,calibrator})} - Cq_{(\text{ref,calibrator})}$$

2. Normalize the ΔCq of the test sample to the ΔCq of the calibrator:

$$\Delta\Delta Cq = \Delta Cq_{(\text{test})} - \Delta Cq_{(\text{calibrator})}$$

3. Calculate the expression ratio:
   $2^{-\Delta\Delta Cq}$ = normalized expression ratio (*see* **Note 8**).

## 4 Notes

1. Once reconstituted in nuclease-free water, the siRNA is ready for transfection at your choice of final siRNA concentration.
2. Complex formation between the siRNA and transfection reagent requires minimum to untraceable amounts of serum as it may interfere with the reaction. Once the complex has successfully formed, downstream procedure can be carried out in serum-containing medium. Check serum compatibility with your chosen transfection reagent.
3. The recommended cell density for a 6-well plate is $2 \times 10^5$ cells/well; cells must be seeded in antibiotic-free normal growth medium supplemented with fetal bovine serum (FBS).

4. It is not necessary to add or replace transfection reagent complex during the incubation period.
5. Prepare cDNA by first isolating the total RNA from transfected cells using an extraction method of choice. RNA must be of high integrity, and yield should be ≥100 ng/μL.
6. The annealing temperature must be optimized as it will not always be 60 °C for different genes. To identify the optimum annealing temperature, we recommend that you run a 5-point temperature gradient, and select the best one.
7. It is advisable to perform a melt curve analysis at the end of a qPCR run to ensure that the fluorescence signal detected during the experiment was generated from a single amplicon. This is because SYBR binds to any double-stranded DNA in the reaction mixture, which, in addition to the newly synthesized amplicon, may include primer dimers, nonspecific amplification, or other anomalies. During melt curve analysis, the temperature steadily increases from about 60 °C to about 95 °C, denaturing the DNA in the post-reaction mixture. A post-qPCR reaction mixture with a single amplicon will generate a smooth decrease in the fluorescence signal to background levels as the DNA "melts." Generating a single peak indicates that a single amplicon was produced, and this can be further confirmed by observing a single band in gel electrophoresis. Multiple peaks, malformed peaks, or abnormally wide peaks are indicative of additional unwanted products in the post-qPCR reaction mixture.
8. A negative $-\Delta\Delta C_q$, in the $2^{-\Delta\Delta C_q}$, is representative of reduction in gene expression, and a positive $-\Delta\Delta C_q$ often represents an overexpression of the target gene compared to the reference sample.

## References


1. Hammond SM, Caudy AA, Hannon GJ (2001) Post-transcriptional gene silencing by double-stranded RNA. Nat Rev Genet 2:110–119. https://doi.org/10.1038/35052556
2. Agrawal N, Dasaradhi PV, Mohmmed A, Malhotra P, Bhatnagar RK, Mukherjee SK (2003) RNA interference: biology, mechanism, and applications. Microbiol Mol Biol Rev 67: 657–685. https://doi.org/10.1128/mmbr.67.4.657-685.2003
3. Zapletal D, Kubicek K, Svoboda P, Stefl R (2023) Dicer structure and function: conserved and evolving features. EMBO Rep 24:e57215. https://doi.org/10.15252/embr.202357215
4. Vermeulen A, Behlen L, Reynolds A, Wolfson A, Marshall WS, Karpilow J, Khvorova A (2005) The contributions of dsRNA structure to dicer specificity and efficiency. RNA 11:674–682. https://doi.org/10.1261/rna.7272305
5. Ma H, Zhang J, Wu H (2014) Designing Ago2-specific siRNA/shRNA to avoid competition with endogenous miRNAs. Mol Ther Nucleic Acids 3:e176. https://doi.org/10.1038/mtna.2014.27
6. Pratt AJ, MacRae IJ (2009) The RNA-induced silencing complex: a versatile gene-silencing machine. J Biol Chem 284:17897–17901. https://doi.org/10.1074/jbc.R900012200
7. Kim TK, Eberwine JH (2010) Mammalian cell transfection: the present and the future. Anal Bioanal Chem 397:3173–3178. https://doi.org/10.1007/s00216-010-3821-6

8. Lefterova MI, Haakonsson AK, Lazar MA, Mandrup S (2014) PPARγ and the global map of adipogenesis and beyond. Trends Endocrinol Metab 25:293–302. https://doi.org/10.1016/j.tem.2014.04.001
9. Lee M-J, Chen H-T, Ho M-L, Chen C-H, Chuang S-C, Huang S-C, Fu Y-C, Wang G-J, Kang L, Chang J-K (2013) PPARγ silencing enhances osteogenic differentiation of human adipose-derived mesenchymal stem cells. J Cell Mol Med 17:1188–1193. https://doi.org/10.1111/jcmm.12098

# Chapter 13

# Freezing and Thawing of Adipose-Derived Stromal/Stem Cells (ASCs)

**Ladislaus Tapiwa Adam, Michael S. Pepper, and Melvin A. Ambele**

## Abstract

Adipose-derived stromal/stem cells (ASCs) have generated great interest both with regard to research and their potential applications in translational clinical sciences. ASCs are often required for use at a later time relative to the time at which they were harvested. This requires appropriate conditions and procedures for storage and retrieval of these cells as needed. This protocol describes cryopreservation and thawing of ASCs without compromising the viability of the stored cells.

**Key words** Adipose-derived stem cells (ASCs), Cryopreservation, Thawing, DMSO, Freezing medium, Dulbecco's Modified Eagle Medium

## 1 Introduction

Adipose-derived stromal/stem cells (ASCs) have found applications in clinical research and regenerative medicine where they are being investigated for use in the treatment of diseases such as acute myocardial infarction, liver cirrhosis, and stroke [1–3]. ASCs may be required in large numbers and often at times well beyond the time of harvest [4]. As a result, they may require storage or preservation for transport and future use. Cryopreservation is used to store ASCs and preserve their viability and multilineage differentiation potential [5]. ASC preservation techniques make use of cryoprotectants like dimethyl sulfoxide (DMSO), methyl cellulose, and polyvinylpyrrolidone (PVP), among others [6]. Under cryopreservation, ASCs have been reported to retain most of their physiological properties for periods up to 10 years [4]. This chapter describes the protocol for cryopreservation and thawing of ASCs.

Michael S. Pepper and Melvin A. Ambele (eds.), *Adipogenesis: Methods and Protocols*, Methods in Molecular Biology, vol. 2938, https://doi.org/10.1007/978-1-0716-4607-6_13,

## 2 Materials

### 2.1 Adipose-Derived Stromal/Stem Cells

Human adipose-derived stromal/stem cells (ASCs) that need to undergo freezing or thawing could be:

1. Human adipose-derived stromal/stem cells (ASCs) that have been freshly isolated from either lipoaspirates or solid fat tissue samples.
2. ASCs recently detached from cell cultures that need to be stored for future use.
3. Cryopreserved ASCs for thawing and use in research or other applications.

### 2.2 Equipment

1. Laminar air flow cabinet (BSL II).
2. Centrifuge.
3. Vacuum aspirator.
4. A −80 °C freezer.
5. Liquid nitrogen storage dewar.
6. Flow cytometer.

### 2.3 General Materials and Supplies

1. Pipettes and pipette tips.
2. Centrifuge tubes.
3. Cryovials.
4. Cell freezing containers.
5. Dulbecco's Modified Eagle Medium (DMEM).
6. Penicillin/streptomycin (Pen/Strep).
7. Fetal bovine serum (FBS).
8. Phosphate-buffered saline (PBS).
9. Dimethyl sulfoxide (DMSO).

### 2.4 Media Stock Solution Preparation

Complete DMEM medium (500 mL): Add 50 mL of fetal bovine serum (10% vol/vol) and 10 mL of Pen/Strep (2% vol/vol) to 440 mL of DMEM medium. Gently swirl the bottle a few times to ensure proper mixing, and store the media at temperatures between 4 and 8 °C.

Cryopreservation medium (3 mL): To 2.7 mL of complete DMEM medium, add 300 μL of DMSO (10% final concentration) (*see* **Note 1**).

## 3 Methods

### 3.1 Freezing Cells

1. Determine the number of cells using any appropriate cell counting technique, and resuspend the cells in cryopreservation medium to a final concentration of $1 \times 10^6$ cells/mL (*see* **Note 2**).
2. Immediately transfer aliquots of 1 milliliter (1 mL) of the cell suspension into well-labelled cryovials; ensure that the labels will not be affected during the freezing and thawing processes.
3. Place cryovials in cell freezing containers, and store in a −80 °C freezer for 24 h (*see* **Note 3**).
4. Transfer the cells in cryovials to a liquid nitrogen dewar for storage in the vapor phase of liquid nitrogen (*see* **Note 4**).

### 3.2 Thawing Cells

1. Pre-warm complete DMEM to 37 °C (place medium container in a 37 °C incubator or water bath for at least 1 h before use).
2. Prefill 50 mL tubes with pre-warmed complete DMEM.
3. Remove the cells from liquid nitrogen dewar, and immediately keep them warm by holding the cryovials between your palms (*see* **Note 5**).
4. Once the frozen cell pellet has thawed into suspension in the cryovials, transfer it into a 50 mL tube containing pre-warmed medium.
5. Centrifuge at 500×*g* for 5 min; then, discard the supernatant leaving behind the cell pellet.
6. Repeat **steps 4** and **5** twice to completely wash away all DMSO from the cells.
7. Resuspend the washed cell pellet in 1 mL of complete medium, and perform cell counts (*see* **Note 6**).

## 4 Notes

1. The cryopreservation medium has to be freshly prepared each time it is used. If cell suspension in complete DMEM is already available, DMSO to a final concentration of 10% can be added directly to the cell suspension.
2. When starting with trypsinized cells, it is recommended to wash the cell suspension twice with either complete DMEM, PBS, or PBS supplemented with 10% FBS (prepared by adding 50 mL of FBS to 450 mL of PBS at pH 7.4), and then perform cell counts.
3. Use freezing containers that support a cooling rate of 1 °C per min.

4. Ensure that cryovials are not in direct contact or immersed in liquid nitrogen.
5. DMSO is cytotoxic to cells; it is important that cells are immediately washed to remove any traces of DMSO. Keeping the frozen cryovial in the palm of your hands facilitates the immediate thawing into suspension of the frozen cells.
6. Following washing, cells are ready for use and can be resuspended in the appropriate medium depending on downstream application. Cell counts can be performed using the Trypan Blue exclusion assay (*see* Chapter 3, **steps 9–12** in Subheading 3.3).

## Acknowledgements

This work was supported by the South African Medical Research Council (Extramural Unit for Stem Cell Research and Therapy) and the University of Pretoria via the Institute for Cellular and Molecular Medicine.

### References

1. Zhao RC (2013) Essentials of mesenchymal stem cell biology and its clinical translation. Springer, Dordrecht
2. Yu G, Wu X, Dietrich MA et al (2015) Yield and characterization of subcutaneous human adipose-derived stem cells by flow cytometric and adipogenic mRNA analyses. Cytotherapy 12:538–546. https://doi.org/10.3109/14653241003649528.Yield
3. Mailey B, Hosseini A, Baker J et al (2014) Adipose-derived stem cells: methods for isolation and applications for clinical use. In: Kioussi C (ed) Stem cells and tissue repair. Humana Press, New York, pp 161–181
4. Shaik S, Wu X, Gimble J, Devireddy R (2018) Effects of decade long freezing storage on adipose derived stem cells functionality. Sci Rep 8: 8162. https://doi.org/10.1038/S41598-018-26546-7
5. Vakhshori V, Bougioukli S, Sugiyama O et al (2018) Cryopreservation of human adipose-derived stem cells for use in ex vivo regional gene therapy for bone repair. Hum Gene Ther Methods 29:269–277. https://doi.org/10.1089/hgtb.2018.191
6. Hunt CJ (2011) Cryopreservation of human stem cells for clinical application: a review. Transfus Med Hemother 38:107. https://doi.org/10.1159/000326623

# Chapter 14

# Isolation and Characterization of Mouse Adipose-Derived Stromal/Stem Cells

Kimberly Thando Peta, Michael S. Pepper, and Melvin A. Ambele

## Abstract

The ability to isolate adipose-derived stromal/stem cells (ASCs) with relative ease has generated a great deal of interest in their potential use for regenerative medicine purposes. ASCs have shown promise in areas such as graft-versus-host disease and wound healing. Murine ASCs (mASCs) can be isolated from various adipose tissue sites. To further explore their therapeutic potential, it is crucial to be able to successfully isolate, expand, and characterize these cells. White adipose tissue (WAT) and brown adipose tissue are the main adipose tissue categories. This chapter presents a protocol for the isolation, expansion, and characterization of mASCs from excised WAT.

**Key words** Mouse adipose-derived stomal/stem cells, Isolation, Expansion, Characterization, Differentiation, Immunophenotype, White adipose tissue

## 1 Introduction

In 2011, the discovery of adipose-derived stromal/stem cells (ASCs), one of the types of mesenchymal stem cells (MSCs), sparked interest in their potential applications in regenerative medicine and tissue engineering [1]. ASCs have been extensively studied and have shown potential in various therapeutic areas such as fibrosis, atrophy, refractory acute graft-versus-host disease, idiopathic thrombocytopenic purpura, and wound healing [2]. In humans, ASCs are obtained from adipose tissue, fat, or liposuction aspirates [3, 4].

Murine ASCs (mASCs) can be isolated from various adipose tissue sites such as anterior subcutaneous, dorsolumbar, inguinal, gluteal, popliteal, omental, and pericardial [5]. There are two main categories of adipose tissue: brown adipose tissue (BAT) and white adipose tissue (WAT) [4–7]. WAT plays a significant role in maintaining energy homeostasis, while BAT, although less abundant

Michael S. Pepper and Melvin A. Ambele (eds.), *Adipogenesis: Methods and Protocols*, Methods in Molecular Biology, vol. 2938,
https://doi.org/10.1007/978-1-0716-4607-6_14,

than WAT, is involved in adaptive thermogenesis and glucose homeostasis [1, 5]. ASCs isolated from WAT display therapeutic potential [8].

In this chapter, we describe a protocol for the isolation, expansion, and characterization of mASCs from inguinal WAT.

## 2 Materials

### 2.1 Reagents and Equipment

1. Sterile scissors and forceps for aseptic dissection of mouse adipose tissue.
2. Sterile nylon mesh (200–250 μm pore size) to filter digested adipose tissue.
3. Heated water bath.
4. Vortex.
5. Centrifuge.
6. Tissue culture flasks.
7. Serological pipettes.
8. Collagenase II.
9. Fetal bovine serum (FBS).
10. Bovine serum albumin (BSA), fatty acid-free.
11. Hanks' balanced salt solution (Hanks' BSS).
12. Glutamine solution.
13. Amphotericin.
14. Penicillin/streptomycin (Pen/Strep).
15. DMEM/F-12 culture medium.
16. Tissue medium (TM): Add 1 mg of BSA in 100 mL of Hanks' BSS to make a 1% BSA solution; then, sterile filter the solution using a 0.22-μm filter, and store at −20 °C for long-term storage.
17. Digestion medium (DM): Weigh out 0.8 mg of collagenase II, and add 1 mL of TM (0.8 mg/mL collagenase II). Sterile filter the solution using a 0.22-micron filter to use immediately (*see* **Note 1**).
18. Use 30 mL of DM to digest adipose tissue from five mice or fewer, and then an additional 5 mL of DM should be added for each additional mouse adipose tissue.
19. Complete culture medium (CCM): Add 100 mL of FBS, 10 mL of Pen/Strep, 5 mL of glutamine, and 1 mL of amphotericin to 384 mL of DMEM/F-12 culture medium.
20. Anti-mouse antibodies: CD45-Brilliant Violet 421 (30-F11), CD90.2-APC (53-2.1), CD31-PE (390), CD29-FITC

(HMb1-1), CD105-PE-C7 (MJ7/18), and CD106-PE-C7 (429).

21. Phosphate-buffered saline (PBS).
22. Dulbecco's Modified Eagle Medium (DMEM).

## 3 Methods

### 3.1 Isolation and Expansion Procedure (Under Sterile Conditions)

1. Place DM in a water bath at 37 °C (*see* **Note 2**).
2. Use a forceps to transfer WAT into a sterile tissue culture dish (*see* **Notes 3**, **4**, and **5**).
3. Gently mince the WAT into small pieces using sterile scissors. The smaller the minced pieces, the better the digestion and the higher the mASC yield.
4. Pour the minced WAT into the DM at 37 °C, and incubate further at 37 °C in the water bath for 40 min. Briefly vortex the mixture every 5 min.
5. Filter the digested tissue through a 200–250-μm-pore-size nylon mesh into a sterile 50 mL falcon tube containing 10–15 mL of CCM (*see* **Note 6**).
6. Centrifuge the mixture at 500×*g* for 7 min.
7. Slowly aspirate the supernatant, leaving behind the pellet that contains mASCs.
8. Resuspend the pellet in an appropriate volume of CCM (8 mL for a T80 flask), and plate it in a culture flask for expansion.
9. Plate isolated ASCs at a seeding density of $5 \times 10^3$ cells/cm$^3$ in 75 cm$^3$ culture flasks (*see* **Note 7**).
10. Place the flasks in a temperature-controlled incubator set at 37 °C and 5% $CO_2$ for continuous cell expansion.

### 3.2 Immunophenotype

1. Add 3 mL of PBS to mASCs in the culture flask, and gently shake to ensure all the cells are washed. Discard the PBS. Repeat this wash step twice to thoroughly rinse the cells (*see* **Note 8**).
2. Add 7 mL of trypsin to the washed cells inside the culture flask.
3. Incubate the flask for 5 min in a 37 °C/5% $CO_2$ incubator, and check to make sure the cells detach from the surface of the flask into suspension.
4. Add an equal volume of CCM (7 mL) to the dissociated cell suspension.
5. Transfer the cell suspension to a 15 mL tube.
6. Centrifuge the cell suspension at 500×*g* for 7 min.
7. Transfer 100 μL of the cell suspension to flow cytometry tubes.

8. Add 5 μL of each antibody to the cells in the tubes, and incubate for 15 min in the dark.
9. Use the following anti-mouse antibodies for staining (*see* **Note 9**):
   - CD45-Brilliant Violet 421 (30-F11).
   - CD90.2-APC (53-2.1).
   - CD31-PE (390).
   - CD29-FITC (HMb1-1).
   - CD105-PE-C7 (MJ7/18).
   - CD106-PE-C7 (429).
10. The cell stained with CD105 should be in a separate tube since this marker has the same fluorochrome as CD106.
11. Visualize and analyze the stained cells using a flow cytometer.

## 4 Notes

1. A fresh solution of DM should be prepared each time just before use to maintain optimal enzymatic activity of the collagenase II.
2. It is important to keep all solutions and media used during the isolation process at a constant temperature of 37 °C to optimize yield.
3. Minimize time: Minimizing the time between WAT harvesting and mASC isolation is critical for optimal results. Time should be minimized to prevent potential molecular changes or decrease in the viability of isolated cells.
4. Maintain sterility: It is essential to maintain strict sterility throughout the procedure. Sterile techniques, including working in a biosafety cabinet, should be followed to prevent contamination and ensure the purity of the isolated mASCs.
5. When extracting WAT from mice, it is crucial to ensure the removal of lymph nodes from WAT. This step is important to minimize potential interference in mASC yield due to the presence of an abundance of immune cells in lymph nodes. Lymph nodes usually appear as small dark brown spots located at the end of blood vessels in WAT.
6. CCM contains FBS, which halts collagenase digestion and protects suspended cells from further collagenase activity.
7. To ensure optimal growth and viability of the mASCs, it is important to change the cell culture media twice a week. Regular medium changes provide the necessary nutrients and maintains a favorable environment for cell expansion.

Monitoring the cells is crucial, once they reach confluence, meaning they have fully covered the surface of the flask, they should be passaged into new flasks to facilitate continuous expansion and proliferation.

8. It is crucial to ensure accurate and effective immunophenotyping of mASCs at passage 3 using a flow cytometer. The proper execution of each step, from washing the cells to analyzing the data, is vital for obtaining reliable and meaningful results.
9. mASCs should be positive for CD29 and CD105, while negative for CD31, CD106, CD45, and CD90.2. Additional markers, such as CD44, CD73, and CD146, have also been utilized for the phenotypic characterization of mASCs [9].

## Acknowledgements

This research was funded by the South African Medical Research Council Self-Initiated Research Grant, Grant/Award Number: A1A982; South African Medical Research Council University Flagship Project (SAMRC-RFA-UFSP-01-2013/STEM CELLS); and the SAMRC Extramural Unit for Stem Cell Research and Therapy. Kimberly Peta acknowledges financial support from the National Research Foundation (NRF) of South Africa through a postgraduate bursary.

### References

1. Tsuji W, Rubin JP, Marra KG (2014) Adipose-derived stem cells: implications in tissue regeneration. World J Stem Cells 6:312–321. https://doi.org/10.4252/wjsc.v6.i3.312
2. Si Z, Wang X, Sun C, Kang Y, Xu J, Wang X, Hui Y (2019) Adipose-derived stem cells: sources, potency, and implications for regenerative therapies. Biomed Pharmacother 114:108765. https://doi.org/10.1016/j.biopha.2019.108765
3. Orbay H, Tobita M, Mizuno H (2012) Mesenchymal stem cells isolated from adipose and other tissues: basic biological properties and clinical applications. Stem Cells Int 2012: 461718
4. Esteve Ràfols M (2014) Adipose tissue: cell heterogeneity and functional diversity. Endocrinol Nutr (English Edition) 61:100–112. https://doi.org/10.1016/j.endoen.2014.02.001
5. Bagchi DP, MacDougald OA (2019) Identification and dissection of diverse mouse adipose depots. J Vis Exp. https://doi.org/10.3791/59499
6. Park A, Kim WK, Bae K-H (2014) Distinction of white, beige and brown adipocytes derived from mesenchymal stem cells. World J Stem Cells 6: 33
7. Huang S-J, Fu R-H, Shyu W-C, Liu S-P, Jong G-P, Chiu Y-W, Wu H-S, Tsou Y-A, Cheng C-W, Lin S-Z (2013) Adipose-derived stem cells: isolation, characterization, and differentiation potential. Cell Transplant 22:701–709
8. Ong WK, Sugii S (2013) Adipose-derived stem cells: fatty potentials for therapy. Int J Biochem Cell Biol 45:1083–1086
9. Maddox JR, Liao X, Li F, Niyibizi C (2009) Effects of culturing on the stability of the putative murine adipose derived stem cells markers. Open Stem Cell J 1:54–61. https://doi.org/10.2174/1876893800901010054

# Chapter 15

# Isolation of Adipose-Derived Mesenchymal Stromal/Stem Cells


## Anastasios Athanasiadis, Melvin A. Ambele, and Michael S. Pepper



## Abstract

Adipose-derived mesenchymal stromal/stem cells (AD-MSCs) offer a promising cell source for regenerative medicine due to their easy accessibility and potential application across a wide range of disorders. This chapter describes a standardized enzymatic isolation protocol to extract AD-MSCs from both solid adipose tissue and lipoaspirate. Adipose tissue samples are initially washed with phosphate-buffered saline (PBS) to remove blood contaminants. Tissue is then digested enzymatically with type I collagenase under controlled temperature and agitation to release the stromal vascular fraction (SVF) containing AD-MSCs. The enzyme activity is neutralized using complete growth medium followed by centrifugation to separate the cell pellet from unwanted material. The resulting cell pellet is resuspended and filtered to eliminate residual tissue fragments. After seeding the cells in culture, AD-MSCs in the SVF are characterized by adherence to plastic and the expression of specific cell surface marker (e.g., CD73, CD90, CD105), confirming their identity. This protocol provides a method for isolating viable AD-MSCs for downstream applications.



**Key words** Mesenchymal stromal/stem cells, Primary cell isolation, Isolation protocol, Enzymatic digestion, Adipose tissue, Stromal vascular fraction


## 1 Introduction

To obtain adipose-derived mesenchymal stromal/stem cells (AD-MSCs) from post-procedural harvested fat tissue, enzymatic digestion and centrifugal separation are employed and yield two distinct fractions: mature adipocytes among undigested connective tissue and the stromal vascular fraction (SVF) [1]. The SVF comprises a heterogenous cell population, including pre-adipocytes, adipocytes, erythrocytes, fibroblasts, vascular smooth muscle cells or pericytes, endothelial cells, resident monocytes, macrophages, lymphocytes, and AD-MSCs [2, 3].

Following isolation, the SVF is seeded into tissue culture dishes or flasks, where cells adhere to the tissue culture plasticware and adopt an elongated (spindle-shaped) morphology, facilitating their purification. Further purification is achieved through culture


Michael S. Pepper and Melvin A. Ambele (eds.), *Adipogenesis: Methods and Protocols*, Methods in Molecular Biology, vol. 2938, https://doi.org/10.1007/978-1-0716-4607-6_15,

processes that include swash steps and medium changes. The remaining adherent cells are now referred to as AD-MSCs. Although the AD-MSC population is less heterogenous than SVF, it is not homogenous.

Mesenchymal stromal/stem cells have the potential to become key players in cell-based therapy due to their unique regenerative and secretory properties. Studies on MSCs have demonstrated their potential in bone regeneration [2], cartilage repair [2], regeneration of musculoskeletal tissues [4], neurogenesis [5], myocardium restoration [6], liver regeneration [7], corneal restoration [8, 9], skin regeneration [10], and more.

## 2 Materials

1. Centrifuge tubes (50 mL).
2. Complete growth medium: DMEM containing 10% fetal bovine serum (FBS) and 2% penicillin/streptomycin (Pen/-Strep). Prepare complete growth medium using the following recipe: 440 mL DMEM, 50 mL FBS, and 10 mL Pen/Strep.
3. Phosphate-buffered saline (PBS) containing 2% Pen/Strep. To prepare PBS, dissolve 10 mg human albumin and 4 mL of 0.5 M EDTA (2 mM final concentration) in 996 mL PBS (pH 7.4). Filter using a 0.22 μm filter, and adjust pH to 7–7.5 using NaCl.
4. Collagenase type 1. Prepare 0.1% collagenase type 1 solution by dissolving 0.1 g in 100 mL of PBS (with 2% Pen/Strep) for tissue digestion; increase recipe proportionally to the required final volume.
5. Red blood cell lysing agent (VersaLyse™).
6. Flow cytometry tubes (5 mL).
7. Cell strainer (70 μm).
8. 0.22 μm bottletop filter or syringe filter.
9. Surgical blade and blade holder.
10. Scissors.
11. Tissue culture dish.
12. VDC Ruby.
13. Flow count beads.
14. T75 or T80 flasks.
15. Incubator.
16. Centrifuge.

## 3 Methods

Adipose-derived stromal/stem cell can be isolated from solid adipose tissue or liquid lipoaspirate.

### 3.1 Solid Adipose Tissue

1. Using sterile scissors, cut a medium-sized piece of adipose tissue, and place it in a 150 mm tissue culture dish. Avoid cutting too close to the skin.
2. Using a sterile blade holder and sterile blade, mince the tissues as finely as possible. The finer the tissue is minced, the easier and more complete the digestion will be later.
3. Transfer the minced tissue into a 50 mL centrifuge tube.
4. Repeat **steps 1–3** until you have processed as much tissue as necessary.

### 3.2 Washing the Tissue

1. Transfer a 25 mL adipose tissue sample into a 50 mL centrifuge tube. Repeat as needed with additional centrifuge tubes until the desired total volume of tissue sample is achieved (*see* **Note 1**).
2. Add 25 mL of PBS containing 2% Pen/Strep to each centrifuge tube, filling each centrifuge tube (50 mL final volume).
3. Centrifuge the tubes at $1700 \times g$ for 3 min (*see* **Note 2**).
4. Aspirate the top oil layer that forms; then, transfer the remaining adipose tissue to a new 50 mL tube, leaving the PBS behind (*see* **Note 3**).
5. Repeat the washing process (**steps 2–4**) of the adipose tissue one or two more times, depending on the extent of blood contamination and oil present within the adipose tissue (a reduction in blood contamination and oil present is desirable).
6. Record both the volume and mass of adipose tissue in each tube.
7. Prepare 0.1% collagenase type 1 solution by dissolving 0.1 g in 100 mL of PBS (with 2% Pen/Strep) for tissue digestion. Ensure you have enough collagenase solution to match the volume of your sample (~25 mL per centrifuge tube) (*see* **Note 4**).
8. Filter the collagenase solution into a new Schott bottle using a 0.22 μm bottletop filter or syringe filter, depending on the total volume being filtered.
9. Add 25 mL of the collagenase solution to each centrifuge tube containing adipose tissue. Incubate the tubes at 37 °C in a rotating incubator for 45–60 min at a medium speed.

10. Centrifuge the tubes at 800×*g* for 5 min. After centrifugation, shake the tubes vigorously to disrupt the cell pellet; then, repeat the centrifugation at 800×*g* for 5 min.
11. Aspirate the digested adipose tissue at the top of the tube. Next, carefully remove the collagenase solution until the volume is reduced to 15 mL (*see* **Note 5**).
12. Shake the remaining cell pellet in the liquid within the centrifuge tube; then, filter the contents through a 70 μm cell strainer to remove tissue debris, reducing the number of tubes required to contain the total volume (*see* **Note 6**).
13. Centrifuge the tubes at 800×*g* for 5 min; then, aspirate and discard all the liquid from the cell pellet.
14. Neutralize the collagenase by adding 5 mL of complete DMEM to each pellet. Mix well by pipetting up and down; then, combine all the pellets into a single 50 mL tube (*see* **Note** 7).
15. Top up the combined cell pellet with PBS (with 2% Pen/-Strep); then, centrifuge at 300×*g* for 5 min. Aspirate the supernatant without disturbing the cell pellet.
16. Resuspend the cell pellet in approximately 20 mL of Versa-Lyse™, and incubate for 10 minutes at room temperature (*see* **Note 8**).
17. After incubation, add 20 mL of PBS (with 2% Pen/Strep); then, centrifuge at 300×*g* for 5 min (*see* **Note 9**).
18. Aspirate the supernatant. Then, add 20 mL of PBS (with 2% Pen/Strep) to the cell pellet, and centrifuge again at 300×*g* for 5 min. If blood contamination persists, repeat the VersaLyse™ **steps 16–18**.
19. Aspirate the supernatant, and resuspend the cell pellet in approximately 20 mL of complete DMEM, which will be your final cell suspension volume.
20. Filter the cell suspension through a 70 μm cell strainer.
21. Count the cells:
    21.1 Mix the final cell suspension and transfer 100 μL to a flow cytometry tube.
    21.2 Add 2 μL of VDC Ruby (a nuclear fluorescent dye) to exclude enucleated cells from the count.
    21.3 Add 100 μL of cell count beads.
    21.4 Measure cells/μL using a flow cytometer.
22. Calculate the total cell number: (cell/μL × μL of final suspension).

23. Plate the cells at 50,000 nucleated cells/cm$^2$ in a T75 or T80 flask. Incubate the flask for 72 h at 37 °C with 5% $CO_2$ (*see* **Note 10**).
24. After 72 h, wash the cultures using PBS (with 2% Pen/Strep) to remove nonadherent cells (via aspiration); then, add 7 mL complete DMEM to feed the cells (*see* **Note 11**).

## 4 Notes

1. Lipoaspirate is typically collected in large cylinders containing both adipose tissue and Ringer's lactate solution. Before proceeding with the isolation procedure, allow the sample to settle until the adipose tissue rises to the top. The time for settlement varies depending on how disturbed the mixture is during handling and transportation. Once settled, carefully transfer only the adipose tissue, leaving behind the Ringer's lactate. If the sample appears runny, distribute it into the centrifuge tubes, and perform an initial centrifugation at 1700×*g* for 3 min before proceeding with the washing steps (**steps 2–4**). This initial spin helps to separate the adipose tissue from any residual liquid in the sample. After centrifugation, fill the 50 mL centrifuge tubes halfway with the adipose tissue, and continue the washing process. Adjust the number of centrifuge tubes based upon your centrifuge capacity.
2. Following centrifugation, the sample will separate into three distinct layers. The bottom layer consists of PBS; the middle layer contains the adipose tissue, and the top layer is composed of oil, which originates from the ruptured adipose cells.

   The primary variables needed to determine the relative centrifugal force [RCF, often expressed in × gravity (*g*)] are the rotor radius and the revolutions per minute.

   (a) Rotor radius (r): This is the distance from the center of the rotor to the position of the sample and is measured in cm.

   (b) Revolutions per minute (rpm): This is the speed at which the rotor spins.

   The formula to calculate the relative centrifugal force is:

$$\mathrm{RCF} = (\mathrm{RPM})^2 \times 1.118 \times 10^{-5} \times \mathrm{r}$$

3. When transferring the adipose tissue to a new tube, use a technique known as "sausaging" to separate the compacted tissue from the blood and PBS. To do this, hold the 50 mL centrifuge tube at a 45° angle, and use a glass pipette to create an air channel at the top of the tube to break the vacuum. Then

while holding a new 50 mL centrifuge tube, slowly pour the compacted adipose tissue into the new tube. This process is similar to the technique used when separating egg whites from yolks.

4. To prepare the collagenase solution, add the powder to a Schott bottle; then, add the required amount of PBS containing 2% Pen/Strep, and mix well. For an isolation involving 16 × 25 mL samples, you will need 400 mL of this solution.
5. During the digestion process, AD-MSCs are located within the adipose tissue. After digestion, the AD-MSCs form a pellet at the bottom of the tube, while the digested adipose tissue and collagenase remain toward the top. This process should result in a near to complete digestion. Take extra care when aspirating the supernatant, as it is possible to inadvertently aspirate the AD-MSC pellet.
6. Filtering the cell suspension can be challenging because the cell strainer may become clogged. To address this, use a sterile Pasteur pipette to aspirate the suspension within the filter up and down. A helpful approach is to set up multiple centrifuge tubes, each with a strainer at the top, and allow gravity to assist in filtering the suspension.
7. Neutralization of collagenase activity is necessary to maximize cell viability for downstream applications.

   Complete DMEM: 440 mL DMEM, 50 mL FBS, 10 mL Pen/Strep.
8. After centrifugation, the pellet may have a reddish color due to the residual red blood cells. The use of VersaLyse™ is to lyse any remaining red blood cells.
9. If the VersaLyse™ solution has successfully lysed all the red blood cells, the pellet will have a creamy white color.
10. Cultures should be named according to the lab's established naming conventions; in our case, we start with P0F0.
11. AD-MSC cultures should be fed twice a week with 7 mL of complete growth medium.

## Acknowledgements

This work was supported by the South African Medical Research Council (Extramural Unit for Stem Cell Research and Therapy) and the University of Pretoria via the Institute for Cellular and Molecular Medicine.

## References


1. Peinado JR, Pardo M, de la Rosa O, Malagón MM (2012) Proteomic characterization of adipose tissue constituents, a necessary step for understanding adipose tissue complexity. Proteomics 12(4–5):607–620. https://doi.org/10.1002/pmic.201100355. Epub 2012 Jan 23. PMID: 22246603
2. Levi B, Longaker MT (2011) Concise review: adipose-derived stromal cells for skeletal regenerative medicine. Stem Cells 29(4):576–582. https://doi.org/10.1002/stem.612. PMID: 21305671; PMCID: PMC3323288
3. Bourin P, Bunnell BA, Casteilla L, Dominici M, Katz AJ, March KL, Redl H, Rubin JP, Yoshimura K, Gimble JM (2013) Stromal cells from the adipose tissue-derived stromal vascular fraction and culture expanded adipose tissue-derived stromal/stem cells: a joint statement of the International Federation for Adipose Therapeutics and Science (IFATS) and the International Society for Cellular Therapy (ISCT). Cytotherapy 15(6):641–648. https://doi.org/10.1016/j.jcyt.2013.02.006. Epub 2013 Apr 6. PMID: 23570660; PMCID: PMC3979435
4. Čamernik K, Barlič A, Drobnič M, Marc J, Jeras M, Zupan J (2018) Mesenchymal stem cells in the musculoskeletal system: from animal models to human tissue regeneration? Stem Cell Rev Rep 14(3):346–369. https://doi.org/10.1007/s12015-018-9800-6. PMID: 29556896
5. Badyra B, Sułkowski M, Milczarek O, Majka M (2020) Mesenchymal stem cells as a multimodal treatment for nervous system diseases. Stem Cells Transl Med 9(10):1174–1189. https://doi.org/10.1002/sctm.19-0430. Epub 2020 June 23. PMID: 32573961; PMCID: PMC7519763
6. Cai L, Johnstone BH, Cook TG, Tan J, Fishbein MC, Chen PS, March KL (2009) IFATS collection: human adipose tissue-derived stem cells induce angiogenesis and nerve sprouting following myocardial infarction, in conjunction with potent preservation of cardiac function. Stem Cells 27(1):230–237. https://doi.org/10.1634/stemcells.2008-0273. PMID: 18772313; PMCID: PMC2936459
7. Yang X, Meng Y, Han Z, Ye F, Wei L, Zong C (2020) Mesenchymal stem cell therapy for liver disease: full of chances and challenges. Cell Biosci 27(10):123. https://doi.org/10.1186/s13578-020-00480-6. PMID: 33117520; PMCID: PMC7590738
8. Mittal SK, Omoto M, Amouzegar A, Sahu A, Rezazadeh A, Katikireddy KR, Shah DI, Sahu SK, Chauhan SK (2016) Restoration of corneal transparency by mesenchymal stem cells. Stem Cell Rep 7(4):583–590. https://doi.org/10.1016/j.stemcr.2016.09.001. Epub 2016 Sept 29. PMID: 27693426; PMCID: PMC5063582
9. Alió Del Barrio JL, El Zarif M, de Miguel MP, Azaar A, Makdissy N, Harb W, El Achkar I, Arnalich-Montiel F, Alió JL (2017) Cellular therapy with human autologous adipose-derived adult stem cells for advanced keratoconus. Cornea 36(8):952–960. https://doi.org/10.1097/ICO.0000000000001228. PMID: 28486314
10. Bian D, Wu Y, Song G, Azizi R, Zamani A (2022) The application of mesenchymal stromal cells (MSCs) and their derivative exosome in skin wound healing: a comprehensive review. Stem Cell Res Ther 13(1):24. https://doi.org/10.1186/s13287-021-02697-9. PMID: 35073970; PMCID: PMC8785459

# Chapter 16

# Isolation and Purification of Adipocyte-Derived Extracellular Vesicles (AdEVs) Using Size-Exclusion Chromatography

**Thabiso Eric Motaung**

## Abstract

Adipocyte-derived extracellular vesicles (AdEVs), like other types of extracellular vesicles (EVs), are released from their donor parental cells in varying sizes and large quantities. During this process, diverse cargos are often internalized in the lumen or covalently attached on the surface of these EVs, allowing for their horizontal transfer from adipocytes to non-adipocyte cells. Hence, AdEVs can promote the ability of adipocytes to remodel the tumor microenvironment in cancers affecting, among others, breast and colon tissues by acting as mediators of cell-to-cell communication through the release of bioactive molecules. Cancer-associated adipocytes, for instance, can promote tumor growth, metastasis, and therapeutic resistance by secreting AdEVs carrying oncogenic microRNAs, cytokines, and chemokines, which interact with signaling pathways (e.g., JAK/STAT3 and PI3K/AKT) that lead to tumor formation and cancerous behavior. As the importance of EVs in these processes rapidly gains attention, a reliable method of isolating AdEVs also becomes highly essential. Therefore, this chapter describes the use of size-exclusion chromatography given its ability to preserve vesicle integrity and achieve high sample purity.

**Key words** Adipogenesis and cancer, Adipocyte-derived extracellular vesicles (EVs), EV isolation, Obesity, Size-exclusion chromatography, Tumor microenvironment

## 1 Introduction

Extracellular vesicles (EVs) include exosomes, microvesicles, apoptotic bodies, and oncosomes, all of which can be generated when a eukaryotic cell membrane buds either inwardly or outwardly from the parent cell [1]. These nanoparticles are biologically active constituents, among which proteins, lipids, and microRNAs (miRNAs) can be disseminated between various cell types including adipocytes and tumor cells (Fig. 1). The EV-mediated biological exchange of molecules between cells can impact the behavior and overall response of those on the receiving end. This process makes EVs

Michael S. Pepper and Melvin A. Ambele (eds.), *Adipogenesis: Methods and Protocols*, Methods in Molecular Biology, vol. 2938, https://doi.org/10.1007/978-1-0716-4607-6_16,

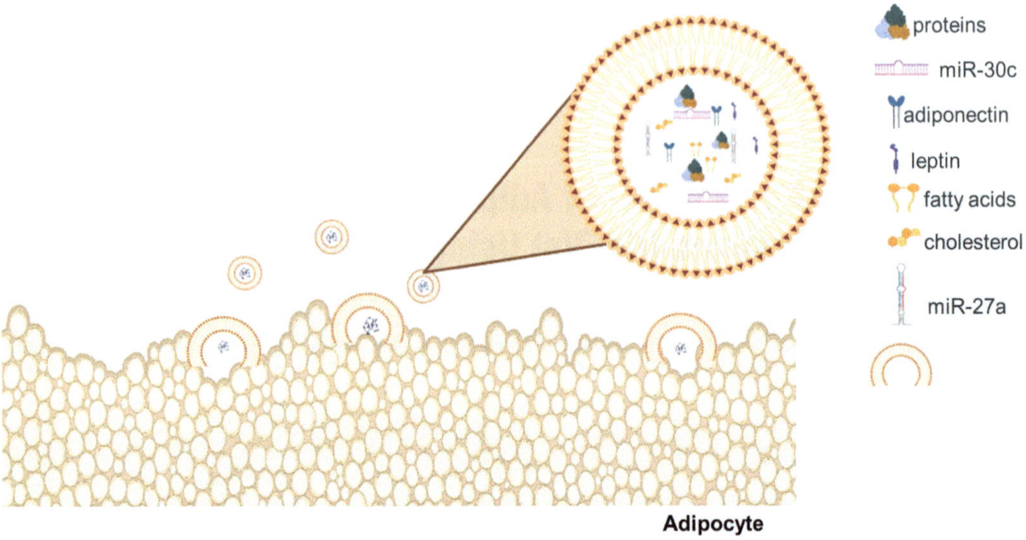


**Fig. 1** A schematic representation depicting an adipocyte releasing extracellular vesicles (adipocyte-derived EVs or AdEVs) along with their molecular cargos, including proteins, microRNAs (miR-30c and miR-27a), adiponectin, leptin, fatty acids, and cholesterol. As illustrated in the magnified view, the various bioactive molecules are delimited by a lipid bilayer, ensuring that they are transferred between cells during intercellular communication and can influence the differentiation and function of target cells.

effective contributors to the overall biological makeup of tissues, influencing how they respond to surroundings.

EVs are also essential in the establishment and maintenance of the tumor microenvironment (TME) through regulating the interaction between tumor cells and their surroundings [2, 3]. However, the association of EVs with factors linking obesity to tumor progression (e.g., secretion of pro-inflammatory cytokines, increased availability of free fatty acids and glucose, elevated levels of pro-angiogenic factors, and secretion of adipokines) was largely unnoticed until in recent years.

Adipogenesis—the process of generating new adipocytes (fat cells)—is one of the most important ways through which metabolic and pathological processes can be modulated [4]. During this process, adipocyte-derived EVs (AdEVs), depending on the physiological or pathological state of the tissue, can influence the differentiation and function of adipocytes by mediating the exchange of bioactive molecules to precursor cells (preadipocytes) and surrounding cells (Fig. 1). AdEVs have accordingly gained much attention in recent years for their role in cancer development, especially where they serve in the cellular interchange of lipids, proteins, and nucleic acids between tumor, stromal, and immune cells (Fig. 1) [5–7]. This can promote cancer cell survival and proliferation [8], leading to a tumor-friendly environment and therefore linking obesity with higher cancer risk and poorer outcomes in several obesity-related cancers.

EVs are therefore influential at the tumor–adipose tissue interface where they can promote the pro-tumorigenic activity of cancer-associated adipocytes (CAAs) (i.e., adipocytes in the TME), supporting cancer growth, invasion, and resistance to therapies [2]. In addition to EVs, CAAs secrete adipokines such as interleukin-6 (IL-6) and leptin, which may enhance cancer cell proliferation, invasion, and metastasis [9]. In breast cancer, these molecules drive cancer progression through pathways such as the Janus kinase and signal transducer and activator of transcription 3 (JAK/STAT3) pathway, promoting cancer cell proliferation and survival [10]. Adipocytes also contribute to drug resistance in cancer through the secretion of AdEVs carrying specific miRNAs and proteins, as indicated in Fig. 1 [6, 11–13]. This may alter the metabolic profile of cancer cells, making them more resistant to chemotherapy [12]. AdEV-associated cargos are also involved in energy metabolism [14, 15], allowing these vesicles to cause cancer cells to withstand chemotherapy-related stresses and continue proliferating under chemical treatment. Collectively, these studies highlight the need to more fully understand the impact of molecular cargos carried by AdEVs on cancer therapy.

Ultracentrifugation is commonly applied for EV isolation; however, it can damage vesicles and co-isolate contaminants. The MISEV2023 (Minimal Information for Studies of Extracellular Vesicles) guidelines, published by the International Society for Extracellular Vesicles, emphasize the need for rigorous isolation and characterization of EVs, ensuring consistency in the isolation procedures, reliability in reporting, and comparability of EV studies [1]. Size-exclusion chromatography (SEC) offers a gentle and efficient method for isolating AdEVs by preserving their structure and biological activity [16, 17]. It may therefore provide a high degree of purity and be ideal for studying the functional roles of AdEVs in cancer [16, 17]. The use of SEC to purify EVs can ensure integrity and reliable isolation and characterization of AdEVs, as recommended by MISEV [1], which is especially important when studying EV-mediated cellular communication and disease processes. In this chapter, a method for isolating AdEVs using SEC is therefore outlined, marking an essential step toward understanding the biology of AdEVs and their role in cancer biology.

## 2 Materials

To successfully purify and characterize AdEVs, the following materials and reagents are needed:

### 2.1 Reagents

1. Phosphate-buffered saline (PBS): Sterilized, with pH adjusted to 7.4.
2. Protease inhibitor cocktail: To avoid proteolysis of the proteinaceous cargos found inside the vesicles during sample preparation (*see* **Note 1**).
3. SEC column: Sepharose CL-2B or commercially available EV isolation kits (e.g., qEV original, Izon).
4. Amicon Ultra-15 filters: 100 kDa molecular weight cutoff for concentrating EVs.
5. Uranyl acetate: For negative staining in TEM.
6. RIPA buffer: For lysing EVs and preparing samples for Western blot analysis.
7. Amicon Ultra-15 filters: 100 kDa molecular weight cut-off, for concentrating EV fractions.
8. Bovine serum albumin (BSA): For blocking generic binding in Western blot and ELISA assays (typically 5% BSA solution in PBS or TBS-T).
9. SDS-PAGE reagents:
   - 4× SDS sample buffer: For denaturing proteins before loading.
   - β-Mercaptoethanol: For reducing protein disulfide bonds.
   - 12% SDS-PAGE gel: For separating proteins by size.
10. Transfer buffer: For protein transfer to PVDF membrane (25 mM Tris, 192 mM glycine, 20% methanol).
11. PVDF membranes: For protein transfer in Western blotting.
12. Primary antibodies: Anti-CD63 (1:1000), anti-CD81 (1:1000), and anti-TSG101 (1:1000).
13. Secondary antibodies: Horseradish peroxidase (HRP)-conjugated anti-mouse or anti-rabbit antibodies (1:5000) for Western blotting and biotinylated secondary antibodies for ELISA (1:500 in PBS-T).
14. Chemiluminescence detection reagents (e.g., ECL substrate): For visualizing protein bands in Western blot.
15. ELISA reagents:
    - Capture antibodies (e.g., anti-CD63, anti-CD81, anti-TSG101).
    - HRP-conjugated streptavidin: For secondary detection in ELISA.
    - TMB substrate (3,3′,5,5′-tetramethylbenzidine): For color development in ELISA.
    - Stop solution: 1 M H2SO4 for stopping the color reaction in ELISA.

16. TBS-T (Tris-buffered saline with Tween-20): For washing in Western blot and ELISA assays.
17. Blocking reagents for ELISA: 1% BSA or 5% nonfat dry milk in PBS-T.
18. BCA protein assay kit: For determining the total protein concentration.

### 2.2 Equipment

1. Centrifuge: Capable of speeds up to 10,000×*g*.
2. Ultracentrifuge: For optional steps involving higher speed sedimentation (not always needed with SEC).
3. Nanoparticle tracking analysis (NTA) device: For size and concentration analysis of EVs.
4. Transmission electron microscope (TEM): For detailed visualization of EV morphology.
5. 0.22 μm filters: To remove debris and large particles before loading samples onto the SEC column.
6. Microcentrifuge tubes (1.5 mL or 2 mL): Sterile polypropylene tubes for collecting and storing EV fractions.
7. Western blotting apparatus:
   - SDS-PAGE gel electrophoresis system: For separating proteins based on size.
   - Power supply unit: For running SDS-PAGE and protein transfer.
   - PVDF membranes: For protein transfer and subsequent immunoblotting.
   - Gel transfer apparatus: For transferring proteins from gel to membrane.
   - Incubation trays: For blocking and antibody incubation.
   - Chemiluminescence detection system: For visualizing protein bands.
   - Gel imager: For capturing and analyzing the Western blot results.
8. ELISA reader:
   - 96-well ELISA plate: For antibody coating and sample incubation.
   - Multichannel pipettes and tips: For accurate addition of reagents.
   - Plate washer or wash bottles: For washing wells between incubation steps.
   - Microplate reader: For measuring absorbance (at 450 nm) after the addition of the substrate.

- Incubator: For maintaining optimal incubation conditions (temperature and time) during ELISA assays.

## 3 Methods

### 3.1 Isolation of Adipocyte-Derived Extracellular Vesicles (AdEVs) Using Size-Exclusion Chromatography (SEC)

Isolation of EVs using SEC is ideal for AdEV purification due to its ability to retain their structural integrity and bioactivity.

1. Collect adipose tissue: Harvest adipose tissue from animal models or human samples. For maximum EV yield, use both subcutaneous and visceral fat depots (*see* **Note 2**).
2. Tissue homogenization: Place the adipose tissue in a cold PBS solution (10 mL PBS per 1 g of tissue) containing a protease inhibitor cocktail (final concentration 1%, typically 100 μL of stock protease inhibitor solution per 10 mL of PBS) to prevent the degradation of sensitive proteins within the EVs (*see* **Note 3**).
3. Homogenize the tissue using a sterile homogenizer until it reaches a consistent slurry.
4. Centrifugation and filtration: Centrifuge the homogenate at 10,000×*g* for 20 min to pellet cellular debris and large organelles.
5. Filter the supernatant through a 0.22 μm filter to eliminate any residual large particles and non-vesicular components.
6. Preparation of the SEC column: Equilibrate the SEC column with room temperature (RT) PBS (20–25 °C) to guarantee its readiness for sample loading (*see* **Note 4**). Sepharose CL-2B or similar columns are widely used for EV isolation but commercial columns (e.g., qEV) are also acceptable (*see* **Note 5**).
7. Loading the sample: Carefully load the sifted sample (supernatant) onto the top of the SEC column. Let the sample pass through the column by gravity flow.
8. Elution: Elute the vesicles by slowly adding RT PBS to the column. Collect fractions at set intervals, typically every 0.5–1 mL using 1.5 mL or 2 mL sterile polypropylene microcentrifuge tubes. The first few fractions are likely to contain EVs, while fractions collected later will contain smaller molecules, such as free proteins and soluble factors.
9. Fraction screening: Test each fraction for EV markers like CD63, CD81, or TSG101 using Western blot analysis or ELISA to confirm the presence of EVs.
10. Pool the fractions that contain EVs for characterization using techniques such as Western blotting, NTA, and TEM, to confirm their identity and purity.

### 3.2 Concentration

After SEC, concentrate the pooled fractions using *Amicon Ultra-15 filters* with a 100 kDa cutoff according to the manufacturer's instructions (*see* **Note 6**). This will facilitate handling of downstream analyses (e.g., TEM, NTA, or proteomic analysis).

### 3.3 Verification of EV Presence Using Western Blot Analysis

1. Protein concentration: Use a protein quantification assay, such as BCA assay, to determine the protein concentration in each EV fraction collected.
2. Particle-to-protein ratio: Next, determine the particle concentration using NTA, and calculate the particle-to-protein ratio (*see* **Note 7**).
3. Lysis buffer: Prepare EV samples by adding a lysis buffer containing RIPA buffer supplemented with protease inhibitors (e.g., PMSF, EDTA, leupeptin) at a 1:100 dilution ratio.
4. Incubation: Incubate the samples on ice for 30 min to ensure complete lysis of vesicles.
5. Centrifugation: Centrifuge the lysates at 14,000×*g* for 15 min at 4 °C to remove insoluble material (e.g., unlysed vesicles or protein aggregates).

### 3.4 SDS-PAGE and Western Blotting

1. Gel preparation: Prepare a 12% SDS-PAGE gel for separating proteins.
2. Loading and running the gel: Mix 20 μg of each protein sample with 4 × SDS sample buffer (containing β-mercaptoethanol) and boil at 95 °C for 5 min.
3. Load the samples onto the gel along with a pre-stained protein ladder.
4. Run the gel at 100 V for 10 min; then, increase to 150 V until the dye front reaches the bottom (approx. 1 h).
5. Transfer the proteins from the gel to a PVDF membrane at 100 V for 90 min in a cold transfer buffer (25 mM Tris, 192 mM glycine, 20% methanol).
6. Blocking: Incubate the membrane in 5% nonfat dry milk (in TBS-T) for 1 h at room temperature.
7. Primary antibody incubation: Incubate the membrane with primary antibodies against CD63 (1:1000), CD81 (1:1000), or TSG101 (1:1000) in 5% milk overnight at 4 °C.
8. Washing: Wash the membrane three times for 10 min each with TBS-T (TBS + 0.1% Tween-20).
9. Secondary antibody incubation: Incubate the membrane with a horseradish peroxidase (HRP)-conjugated secondary antibody (1:5000) in 5% milk for 1 h at room temperature.

10. Washing: Wash the membrane three times for 10 min each with TBS-T.
11. Detection: Detect the protein bands using an enhanced chemiluminescence (ECL) detection system. Visualize using a gel imaging system or X-ray film.
12. The presence of CD63 (53–60 kDa), CD81 (25 kDa), or TSG101 (43 kDa) bands confirms the presence of EVs in the respective fractions (*see* **Note 8**).

### 3.5 Verification of EV Presence Using Enzyme-Linked Immunosorbent Assay (ELISA)

1. Coating: Coat a 96-well ELISA plate with 100 μL of capture antibody (anti-CD63, anti-CD81, or anti-TSG101, 1:200 dilution in PBS), and incubate overnight at 4 °C.
2. Washing: Wash the plate three times with PBS-T (PBS + 0.1% Tween-20).
3. Blocking: Block the wells with 200 μL of 1% BSA in PBS-T for 1 h at room temperature to prevent nonspecific binding.
4. Dilute each EV fraction (e.g., 50 μL per well) to a total volume of 100 μL in PBS-T.
5. Incubate for 2 h at room temperature.
6. Wash the wells three times with PBS-T.
7. Add 100 μL of biotinylated anti-CD63, anti-CD81, or anti-TSG101 antibody (1:500 in PBS-T), and incubate for 1 h at room temperature.
8. Wash the wells three times with PBS-T.
9. Add 100 μL of HRP-conjugated streptavidin (1:1000 in PBS-T), and incubate for 30 min at room temperature.
10. Wash the wells three times with PBS-T.
11. Add 100 μL of TMB substrate (3,3′,5,5′--tetramethylbenzidine) to each well, and incubate for 10–15 min in the dark.
12. Stop the reaction by adding 50 μL of 1 M H2SO4.
13. Measure absorbance at 450 nm using a plate reader.
14. A higher absorbance indicates a greater presence of the target EV markers in the fractions.

## 4 Notes

1. *Protease inhibitor cocktail:* The use of a protease inhibitor cocktail in tissue homogenization minimizes the degradation of EV proteins. The cocktail can either be purchased as a ready-made product or prepared from individual constituents. It typically includes inhibitors for various classes of proteases, such as

serine proteases (e.g., trypsin, chymotrypsin), cysteine proteases (e.g., papain, cathepsins), aspartic proteases (e.g., pepsin), and metalloproteases (e.g., matrix metalloproteinases). Common constituents in a prepared cocktail include PMSF (phenylmethylsulfonyl fluoride), EDTA (ethylenediaminetetraacetic acid), and leupeptin.

2. Obtaining EVs from subcutaneous and visceral samples can increase the overall quantity of EVs to facilitate downstream analyses (e.g., protein and RNA profiling and functional studies) of AdEVs. In addition, this can provide a more complete representation of the entire adipose tissue in terms of a collection of secreted molecules (secretome).
3. The volume ratio of 10 mL of PBS per 1 g of tissue is recommended for effective sample dilution and to maintain appropriate conditions for EV stability during homogenization. Additionally, the 1% protease inhibitor cocktail is optimal to inhibit a broad spectrum of proteases, ensuring minimal degradation of EV-associated proteins.
4. It is recommended to use room temperature PBS (20–25 °C) for equilibrating the SEC column to maintain the best flow rates and bead functionality. Cold PBS (4 °C) is ideal for preserving vesicle integrity; however, it may impact the flow rate and separation efficiency contingent on the type of beads (e.g., Sepharose CL-2B). For this reason, it is best to keep a close eye on flow rate when using cold PBS.
5. Sepharose CL-2B is made up of agarose beads with a pore size and fractionation range (70,000 to 20,000,000 daltons) broad enough for separating large EVs (30–200 nm in size) from smaller molecules such as proteins and nucleic acids. This makes it ideal for the efficient exclusion of smaller impurities while allowing EVs to pass through. qEV columns are more appropriate for repetitive and small-scale use. Since they can be used with great ease, they offer high-throughput EV isolations in standardized EV studies.
6. It is recommended to follow the manufacturer's instructions for centrifugation speeds and volumes when using Amicon Ultra-15 filters. However, for EV-specific applications, monitor the final volume carefully to avoid overconcentration, which can lead to vesicle aggregation. It is recommended to spin at 4000×*g* at 4 °C and include a final wash with 1–2 mL of RT PBS if additional purification is needed to minimize non-vesicular contaminants.
7. Determining the particle-to-protein ratio is an important quality control step to guarantee the enrichment of vesicles relative to free proteins, and it can be valuable before proceeding with Western blot analysis. It is calculated by dividing the

concentration of EV particles (as measured by NTA) by the concentration of total protein (measured using a BCA assay or other protein quantification methods). If the sample has a low particle-to-protein ratio, it could indicate the presence of excess non-vesicular proteins (e.g., albumin or other serum proteins), which can interfere with the detection of EV-specific markers. This can yield false positives and difficulties in confidently confirming the presence of EVs in a sample. A high particle-to-protein ratio is typically $>1 \times 10^{10}$ particles/μg of protein, which is ideal for confirming sample purity since it indicates minimal contamination by free proteins.

8. Due to their abundance, *CD63*, *CD81*, and *TSG101* are widely recognized as the "gold standard" *protein markers* to establish the presence of EVs (exosomes) in a biological sample. CD63 and CD81 are both *tetraspanin proteins*, spanning the cellular membrane four times, and are highly enriched in the membranes of exosomes. On the other hand, TSG101 (tumor susceptibility gene 101 protein) is associated with *endosomal sorting complex required for transport (ESCRT)* system and typically constitutes the cytoplasmic components of exosomes. These protein markers enable EV researchers to reproduce and compare results across multiple studies. Therefore, the use of CD63, CD81, and TSG101 as EV markers during AdEV characterization in Western blotting and ELISA will support the presence of well-defined AdEV populations, thus increasing the confidence for downstream functional studies and ensuring compliance with MISEV.

## Acknowledgement

This work was supported by the Thuthuka Funding Instrument (grant no. 129580) from the South African National Research Foundation (NRF). The author extends gratitude to Melvin Ambele for his valuable comments and suggestions during the writing of this chapter. Special thanks to Francinah Ratsoma for her role in conceptualizing and designing Fig. 1.

### References

1. Welsh JA, Goberdhan DCI, O'Driscoll L et al (2024) Minimal information for studies of extracellular vesicles (MISEV2023): from basic to advanced approaches. J Extracell Vesicles 13:e12404
2. Robado De Lope L, Alcíbar OL, Amor López A et al (2018) Tumour–adipose tissue crosstalk: fuelling tumour metastasis by extracellular vesicles. Philos Trans R Soc B 373:20160485
3. Han L, Lam EW-F, Sun Y (2019) Extracellular vesicles in the tumor microenvironment: old stories, but new tales. Mol Cancer 18:59
4. Luo L, Liu M (2016) Adipose tissue in control of metabolism. J Endocrinol 231:R77–R99
5. Sullivan R, Maresh G, Zhang X et al (2017) The emerging roles of extracellular vesicles as communication vehicles within the tumor

microenvironment and beyond. Front Endocrinol 8:194

6. Maacha S, Bhat AA, Jimenez L et al (2019) Extracellular vesicles-mediated intercellular communication: roles in the tumor microenvironment and anti-cancer drug resistance. Mol Cancer 18:55
7. Kalluri R, McAndrews KM (2023) The role of extracellular vesicles in cancer. Cell 186:1610–1626
8. La Camera G, Gelsomino L, Malivindi R et al (2021) Adipocyte-derived extracellular vesicles promote breast cancer cell malignancy through HIF-1α activity. Cancer Lett 521:155–168
9. Rybinska I, Mangano N, Tagliabue E et al (2021) Cancer-associated adipocytes in breast cancer: causes and consequences. IJMS 22:3775
10. Jung J, Kim NH, Kwon M et al (2023) The inhibitory effect of Gremlin-2 on adipogenesis suppresses breast cancer cell growth and metastasis. Breast Cancer Res 25:128
11. Cao Y (2019) Adipocyte and lipid metabolism in cancer drug resistance. J Clin Invest 129:3006–3017
12. Yang K, Wang L, Cao X et al (2022) The origin, function, distribution, quantification, and research advances of extracellular DNA. IJMS 23:13690
13. Song Y, Na H, Lee SE et al (2024) Dysfunctional adipocytes promote tumor progression through YAP/TAZ-dependent cancer-associated adipocyte transformation. Nat Commun 15:4052
14. Le Lay S, Rome S, Loyer X et al (2021) Adipocyte-derived extracellular vesicles in health and diseases: Nano-packages with vast biological properties. FASEB Bioadv 3:407–419
15. Sandoval-Bórquez A, Carrión P, Hernández MP et al (2024) Adipose tissue dysfunction and the role of adipocyte-derived extracellular vesicles in obesity and metabolic syndrome. J Endocr Soc 8:bvae126
16. Böing AN, Van Der Pol E, Grootemaat AE et al (2014) Single-step isolation of extracellular vesicles by size-exclusion chromatography. J of Extracell Vesicles 3:23430
17. Sidhom K, Obi PO, Saleem A (2020) A review of exosomal isolation methods: is size exclusion chromatography the best option? IJMS 21:6466

# Chapter 17

# Differentiation of Adipose-Derived Stromal/Stem Cells into Osteocytes

**Jamie de Beer and Michael S. Pepper**

## Abstract

Osteogenesis, which refers to the formation of bone tissue, can be studied in vitro to elucidate the mechanisms of bone development, identify key factors and cytokines, and enhance potential regenerative medicine applications in tissue engineering and transplantation. Adipose-derived stromal/stem cells (ASCs) are particularly promising for these studies due to their capacity to differentiate into various mesodermal lineage cells, including osteoblasts. To induce osteogenic differentiation, ASCs are cultured in a complete growth medium (CGM) supplemented with β-glycerophosphate, ascorbate-2-phosphate and dexamethasone over a period of at least 3 weeks. Osteogenic differentiation can be assessed through the deposition of hydroxyapatite, a key component of mineralized bone matrix, and the activity of alkaline phosphatase, an enzyme crucial for matrix calcification. This study provides a protocol for differentiating ASCs into osteoblasts using osteogenic differentiation medium (ODM) and evaluating the differentiation using Alizarin Red S (ARS) staining and alkaline phosphatase (ALP) assays. The methodology includes the preparation of CGM and ODM, as well as the specific procedures for ARS staining and ALP activity assays. The ARS staining involves fixation of cells, staining, and quantification of hydroxyapatite deposition, while the ALP assay measures enzyme activity. Both assays are normalized to cell counts, determined through DAPI staining and microscopic analysis. The results of these assays are intended to provide an accurate evaluation of osteogenic differentiation efficiency in ASCs.

**Key words** Osteogenesis, Adipose-derived stem cells, Evaluation of osteogenesis, Alizarin Red S assay, Alkaline phosphate assay

## 1 Introduction

Osteogenesis, which refers to the process of bone tissue formation, can be studied in vitro to increase our understanding of osteogenesis, investigate the key factors and cytokines involved, and develop scaffolds for regenerative medicine, tissue engineering, and transplantation [1]. Adipose-derived stromal/stem cells (ASCs) are known for their ability to differentiate into various cell types originating from the mesodermal layer, including osteoblasts [1]. To effectively induce osteogenic differentiation, ASCs are cultured in

Michael S. Pepper and Melvin A. Ambele (eds.), *Adipogenesis: Methods and Protocols*, Methods in Molecular Biology, vol. 2938, https://doi.org/10.1007/978-1-0716-4607-6_17,

complete growth medium (CGM) that has been enriched with β-glycerophosphate, ascorbate-2-phosphate, and dexamethasone for at least 3 weeks.

The success of osteogenic differentiation can be evaluated by either looking at the amount of hydroxyapatite deposition or by looking at the level of alkaline phosphate activity. Hydroxyapatite is the main compound found in mineralized bone extracellular matrix, and therefore the more hydroxyapatite, the more successful the osteogenic differentiation was [2]. The enzyme alkaline phosphatase plays a key role in matrix calcification [3].

Here, we demonstrate a method to differentiate ASCs into osteoblasts and to evaluate the success of the osteogenic differentiation. The isolated ASCs are differentiated into osteoblasts by the addition of three compounds, namely, *β*-glycerophosphate, ascorbate-2-phosphate, and dexamethasone [4]. The success of osteogenesis is then measured through ARS and ALP assays.

## 2 Materials

### 2.1 Complete Growth Media (CGM)

Remove 60 mL of DMEM from 500 mL stock DMEM solution. Add 50 mL of FBS thawed at 37 °C Add 10 mL Pen/Strep. Mix the CGM well by inverting the bottle a few times, and filter using a 70 μm filter before use. CGM can be filtered using a 70 μm cell strainer. CGM should be refrigerated at 2–8 °C.

### 2.2 Osteogenic Differentiation Medium (ODM)

1. Ascorbate-2-phosphate (100 mM): Weigh 161.025 mg of ascorbate-2-phosphate, and add to 5 mL of distilled water in a 15 mL tube.
2. *β*-Glycerophosphate: Weigh 6 mg of *β*-glycerophosphate, and add to 2 mL of DMEM. Filter the solution through a 0.2 μm syringe filter.
3. Dexamethasone (1 mM): Weigh 3.92 mg of dexamethasone, and add to 10 mL of 100% ethanol in a 15 mL tube.
4. ODM (working solution): Add 776.25 μL of 100 mM ascorbate-2-phosphate, 1 mL of the *β*-glycerophosphate stock solution, and 0.5 μL of 1 mM dexamethasone into a 500 mL glass bottle. Add CGM to a final volume of 500 mL. Filter the ODM before use using a 70 μm cell strainer.

### 2.3 Phosphate-Buffered Solution (PBS) (2% Penicillin–Streptomycin (Pen/Strep))

1. Weigh 20 g of 68 mM of sodium chloride, 1 g of 2.6 mM of potassium chloride, 5.75 g of 8.1 mM of sodium phosphate dibasic, and 1 g of 1.5 mM of potassium phosphate monobasic. Add the powders to a 5 L bottle. Add 4.5 L of distilled water to the 5 L bottle with powders. Drop a magnetic stirrer into the solution in the bottle. Place the bottle on a magnetic stirrer plate to mix the solution for approximately 20 min or until all powder is dissolved.

2. Adjust the pH to 7.4. To increase the pH, use 1 M of NaOH, and to decrease the pH, use 1 M of HCl.
3. Adjust the volume with distilled water to a final volume of 5 L.
4. Autoclave the PBS solution.
5. To make 500 mL of PBS (2% Pen/Strep) solution, add 10 mL Pen/Strep to 490 mL autoclaved PBS.

### 2.4 Paraformaldehyde (4%)

1. Add 350 mL of 1× PBS to a suitable bottle on a stir plate in a well-ventilated hood. Heat the solution while stirring to approximately 60 °C. Take care that the solution does not boil (*see* **Note 1**).
2. Weigh 20 g of paraformaldehyde powder, and add the powder to the heated PBS solution. Slowly raise the pH by adding 1 N NaOH dropwise from a pipette until the solution clears (*see* **Note 2**).
3. Adjust the pH to between 6.9 and 7.2 with either 1 M NaOH or 1 M HCl.
4. Add 1× PBS to the solution to make it up to 500 mL.
5. Once the paraformaldehyde is completely dissolved, the solution should be cooled and filtered using a filter paper.
6. The solution can be aliquoted and frozen or stored at 2–8 °C for up to 1 month.

### 2.5 Alizarin Red S (ARS) Staining Solution

1. ARS staining solution (2%w/v): Weigh 2 g of ARS staining powder into a 50 mL tube, and add 50 mL of distilled water.
2. Mix the solution well by vortexing the tube.
3. Filter the solution before use by using filter paper.

### 2.6 Alizarin Red S (ARS) Staining Solution (4 mM)

1. Weigh 2.88 mg of ARS powder in a 2 mL tube, and add 2 mL of distilled water to the powder.
2. Mix the solution well by vortexing the tube.
3. Filter the solution before use using a syringe filter (0.2 μm).

### 2.7 Acetic Acid (10% V/V)

Add 1 mL acetic acid to 9 mL of distilled water.

### 2.8 Ammonium Hydroxide (10% V/V)

Add 4 mL of 25% ammonium hydroxide to 6 mL distilled water.

### 2.9 Alkaline Phosphatase (ALP) Buffer (10× Solution)

50 mM 4-nitrophenylphosphate (weigh 0.548 g, and add to 50 mL of distilled water), 5 mM MgCl hexahydrate (weigh 0.05 g, and add to 50 mL of distilled water), 10% Triton X-100, 500 mM Tris–HCl (weigh 3.94 g, and add to 50 mL of distilled water; pH of 9.5). Store the stock solutions at −20 °C until needed.

### 2.10 ALP Buffer (1× Solution)

Add 1 mL of 10× 4-nitrophenylphosphate stock solution, 1 mL of the 10× MgCl hexahydrate stock solution, 1 mL of the 10× Tris–HCl stock solution, and 10 μL of the Triton X-100 stock solution. Add distilled water to a final volume of 10 mL.

## 3 Methods

### 3.1 Osteogenic Differentiation of ASCs

1. Seed ASCs in 6-well culture dish at 5000 cells/cm$^2$, and maintain cells with CGM (2 mL per well) until the cells reach 70–80% confluency.
2. Once a confluency of 70–80% has been reached, replace the CGM with 2 mL ODM. Include a negative control by maintaining cells in CGM (*see* **Note 3**).
3. ODM and CGM are replaced every 2–3 days until the day of termination (*see* **Note 4**).

### 3.2 Assessment of Osteogenic Differentiation Using Alizarin Red S (ARS) Staining Assay

1. Remove CGM or ODM, and wash cells with PBS (2% Pen/-Strep). To wash cells, simply remove the CGM/ODM; add 2 mL of PBS per well, and then remove the PBS again.
2. Fix the cells by adding 2 mL of paraformaldehyde (4% w/v), and incubate for 15 min at room temperature.
3. Wash cells with PBS (2% Pen/Strep) (**step 1**).
4. Add 2 mL of ARS staining solution (2% w/v) to the wells, and incubate the cells for 10 min at room temperature.
5. Remove the unincorporated staining solution by aspirating the liquid, and wash the cells four times with PBS (2% Pen/Strep) (**step 1**).
6. Remove the excess PBS by incubating the plate at a 30° angle for 30 min, and then remove the excess PBS.
7. Air-dry the plates in the dark overnight, and visualize the stained monolayer using a light microscope.

### 3.3 Standard Curve for ARS Staining Assay

1. Perform a series of 1:1 serial dilutions (from 4 mM down to 0.0625 mM) by preparing eight 2 mL tubes. In tubes 2–7, add 1 mL of distilled water. In tube 1, add the filtered 4 mM ARS solution; add 1 mL of tube 1 into tube 2, and mix the solution by vortexing. Again, take 1 mL of tube tube and add it to tube 3 and mix by vortexing. Continue with this serial dilution until you reach tube 7. Tube 8 should just be distilled water as this will serve as our blank. Aliquot 200μL of each tube into a separate well of a 96-well plate (opaque-walled, transparent-bottomed plate), and measure the optical density of each concentration as well as the blank (tube 8) on a spectrophotometer at 405 nm. Perform this in triplicate.

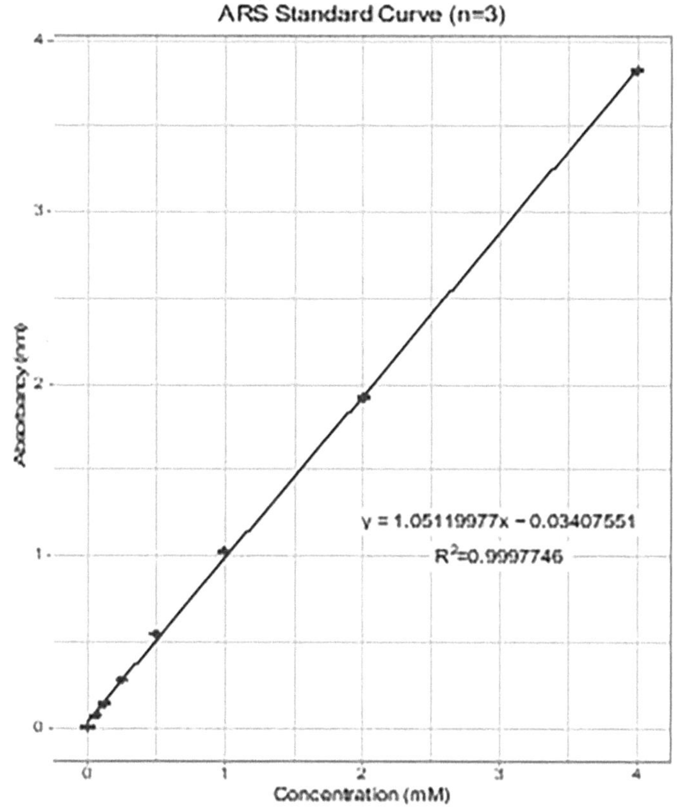


**Fig. 1** ARS standard curve. Standard curve displaying the equation $y = 1.05119977x - 0.03407551$ used to calculate the concentration of ARS

2. Adjust the standard curve optical density (OD) values for background interference by subtracting the average OD reading of the blanks from the OD readings of the standards.
3. Draw up a standard curve by plotting the absorbance (405 nm) $OD405_{nm}$ readings against the ARS concentrations (Fig. 1).

#### 3.4 Quantifying the ARS Staining Assay

1. Extract the incorporated ARS stain by adding 2 mL of acetic acid (10%v/v) to each well, and incubate for 30 min at room temperature.
2. Add 200 μL of ammonium hydroxide (10%v/v) to each well to stop the extraction reaction.
3. Transfer an aliquot of 100 μL of each into a well of a 96-well plate (opaque-walled, transparent-bottomed plate), and measure the OD values at 405 nm and 650 nm (reference) using a spectrophotometer.
4. Determine the ARS concentration of each respective sample by extrapolating the concentration from the ARS standard curve.

### 3.5 Assessment of Osteogenic Differentiation Using Alkaline Phosphatase (ALP) Assay

1. Remove CGM or ODM, and wash cells with PBS (2% Pen/Strep).
2. Fix the cells by adding 2 mL of paraformaldehyde (4% w/v), and incubate for 15 min at room temperature.
3. Wash cells with 2 mL of PBS (2% Pen/Strep) (*see* **step 1** in Subheading 3.2).
4. Add 2 mL of ALP buffer and incubate for 60 min at 37 °C.
5. Transfer an aliquot of 100 μL into a well of a 96-well plate (opaque-walled, transparent-bottomed plate), and measure the OD values at 405 nm and 650 nm (reference) using a spectrophotometer.

### 3.6 Determining Cell Counts for Normalization of ARS and ALP Assays

1. Aspirate the remaining liquid from the assays, and wash the cells with PBS (2% Pen/Strep).
2. Add 2 mL of PBS (2% Pen/Strep) and 1 μL of DAPI (0.02 μg/mL in molecular $H_2O$) into each well, and incubate for 5 min.
3. Capture images using a fluorescent microscope (filter set 49; excitation, green 365; emission, bandpass filter 445/50).
4. Capture five fields of vision per well to obtain a representative cell count (Fig. 2).
5. Determine the area of the field (A = length × width) of vision using a calibrated scale bar.
6. Open .tiff files in ImageJ.
7. Adjust the brightness and the contrast of images (Figs. 3a, c).
8. Convert the image into an 8-bit image, and adjust the threshold to "black and white" (Fig. 3d).

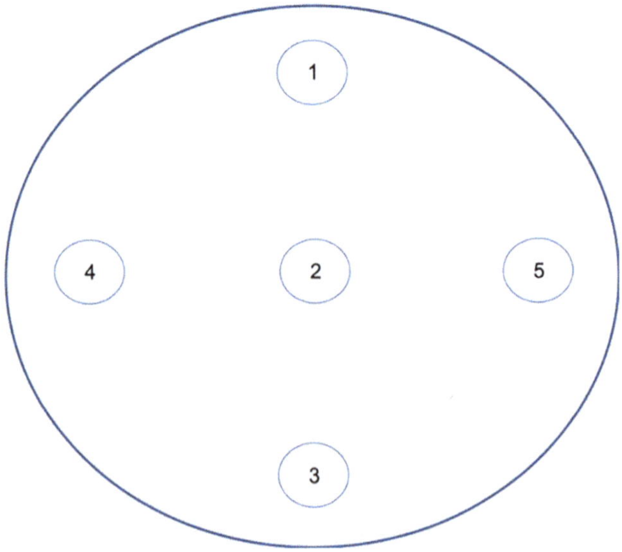


**Fig. 2** Schematic illustration of the approximate position of the fields of visions used to calculate a representative cell count per well

9. Convert the image into a mask using the binary option (Menu: Process > Binary > Convert to Mask) (Fig. 3e).
10. Separate out the connected particles by applying watershed to the image (Menu: Process > Binary > Watershed).
11. Analyze particles/nuclei using the count function under the Analyze menu (Menu: Analyze > Analyze particles). Exclude everything less than 200-pixel units (Fig. 3f–h).
12. Manually assess counted particles/nuclei as cells close to each other were sometimes identified (called) as a single cell. In these cases, manual adjustments are made to the cell counts (Fig. 3i–j).
13. Determine the approximate cell count per well using the following formula:

$$\text{Approximate cell count} = \frac{\text{Average cells from the 5 representative images} \times 9.6\ \text{cm}^2}{\text{Area of field of vision}} \quad (1)$$

**Formula used to calculate the approximate cell count in each well**

### 3.7 Normalization of ARS and ALP Assays

1. Using the cell counts of each well, normalize the concentration of ARS/ALP to the number of cells per well with the following formula:

$$\text{Normalization} = \frac{\text{OD value or Concentration}}{\text{Cell number}} \times \text{Value} \quad (2)$$

**Formula to normalize ARS/ALP concentration to the number of cells per well**

## 4 Notes

1. When heating the paraformaldehyde solution, take care that the solution does not boil as this will change the concentration of the solution.
2. The powder will not immediately dissolve. As the pH of the solution rises, the solution will start to dissolve.
3. It is important to include a negative control to have a baseline reading for assay.
4. The day of termination can vary depending on the source of growth factors. In this case, if the source is FBS, then the optimal day of termination is 28 days. When human alternatives are used, such as pooled human platelet lysate or platelet rich plasma, then the optimal termination day is day 21.

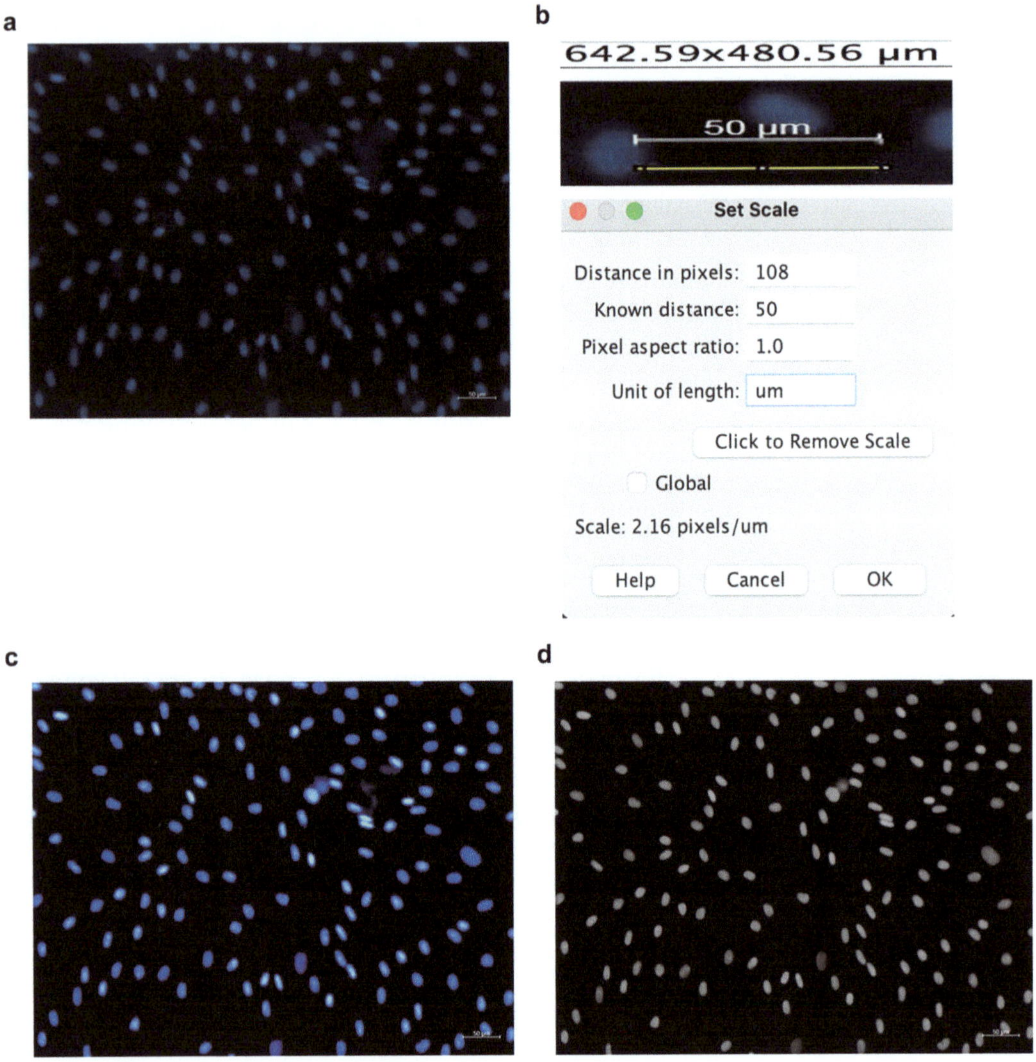


**Fig. 3** A summary of the steps followed to obtain an approximate cell count per well using ImageJ software (**a**). The original image captured (**b**). The scale was calibrated by measuring the scale bar to determine the number of pixels, setting the known distance and entering the correct units. These parameters were all used to calculate the area of the field of vision displayed by the software in the top left-hand corner, e.g., 642.59 × 480.56 μm (**c**). The brightness of the images was adjusted to improve the resolution of the nuclei (**d**). The image was converted to an 8-bit image (**e**). Threshold was adjusted to "B&N" (**f**). The image was analyzed to determine the number of nuclei per field of vision (**g**). The nuclei count as determined by the ImageJ software (**h**). Images were manually assessed, and incorrect calling of events (nuclei), such as the scale bar counted as a nucleus (**i**) or nuclei in close proximity counted as a single event, was corrected (**j**).

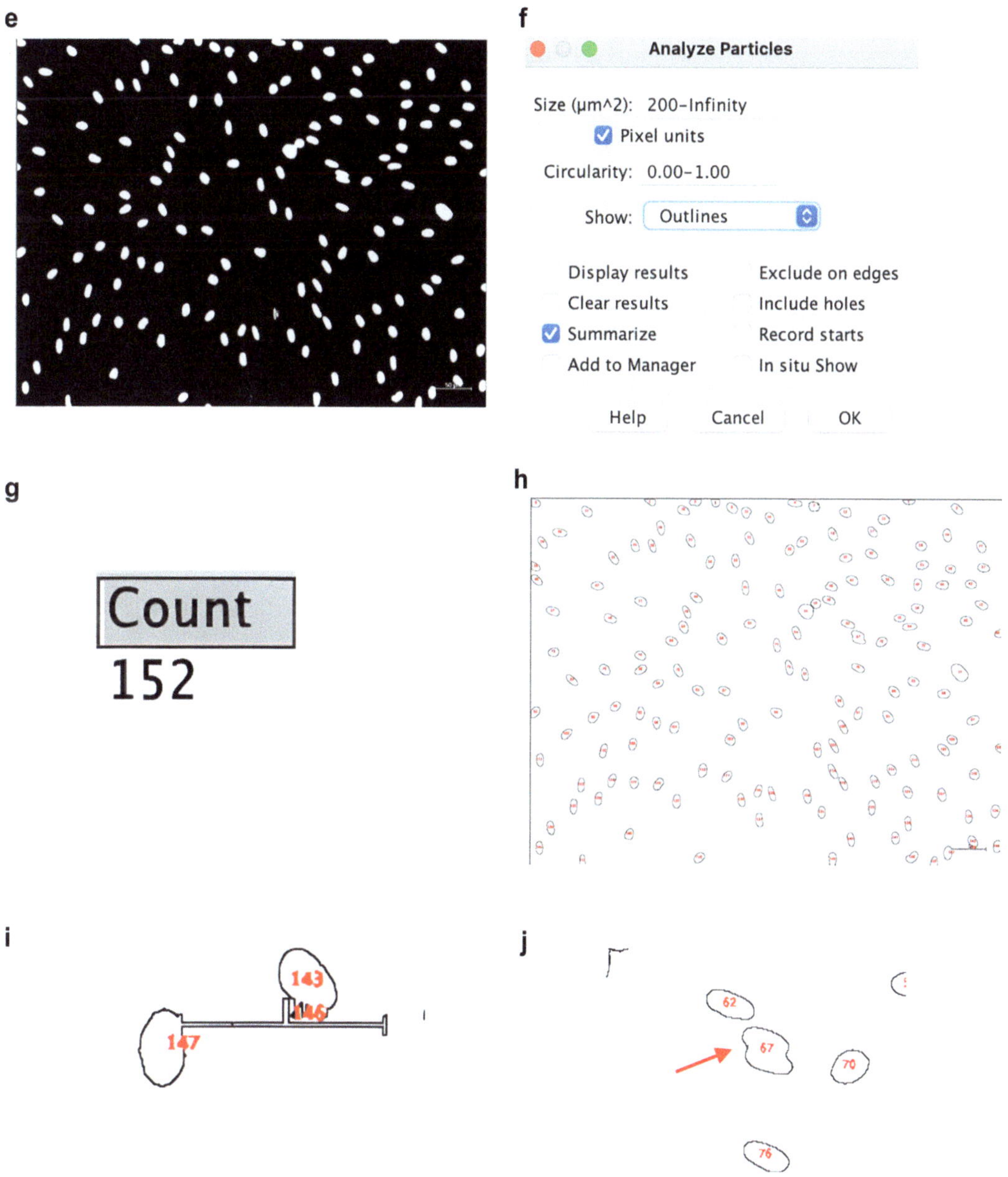


Fig. 3 (continued)

## Acknowledgements

This work was supported by a grant to MSP from the South African Medical Research Council (Extramural Unit for Stem Cell Research and Therapy), the University of Pretoria via the Institute for Cellular and Molecular Medicine, and a postgraduate student bursary to JdB.

## References

1. Wei X, Yang X, Han ZP et al (2013) Mesenchymal stem cells: a new trend for cell therapy. Acta Pharmacol Sin 34:747–754
2. Miklos AC, Li C, Sorrell CD et al (2011) An upper limit for macromolecular crowding effects. BMC Biophys 4. https://doi.org/10.1186/2046-1682-4-13
3. Nishimura I, Hisanaga R, Sato T et al (2015) Effect of osteogenic differentiation medium on proliferation and differentiation of human mesenchymal stem cells in three-dimensional culture with radial flow bioreactor. Regen Ther 2:24–31. https://doi.org/10.1016/j.reth.2015.09.001
4. Li H, Pan S, Xia P et al (2020) Advances in the application of gold nanoparticles in bone tissue engineering. J Biol Eng 14:14

# Chapter 18

# Differentiation of Mesenchymal Stromal/Stem Cells from Induced Pluripotent Stem Cells

**Alex Leah Marais, Murray Glen Logan, Juanita Mellet, Melvin A. Ambele, and Michael S. Pepper**

## Abstract

Mesenchymal stromal/stem cells (MSCs) possess unique immunomodulatory and regenerative properties, making them ideal candidates for addressing a variety of disorders. With an increasing number of clinical trials, reliable sources are needed to obtain sufficient cell numbers and to circumvent inherent limitations associated with primary cells. Induced pluripotent stem cells (iPSCs) can be differentiated into various somatic cell types and are able to proliferate indefinitely in culture. Differentiation of iPSCs presents a viable alternative in order to create target cell types for both proof-of-concept research and therapeutic applications. In this chapter, we present a protocol to derive MSC-like cells from iPSCs as well as methods of characterizing these cells.

**Key words** Induced pluripotent stem cells, Mesenchymal stromal/stem cells, Differentiation, Immunophenotyping, Cell therapy

## 1 Introduction

Stem cells are undifferentiated cells with the potential to differentiate into a variety of cell types and have been recognized as a promising cell source in treating degenerative and other disorders [1]. Mesenchymal stromal/stem cells (MSCs) were initially derived from bone marrow aspirates, although a number of alternative sources have also been identified including fat, dental pulp, and epidermal and embryonic tissues [2]. MSCs are multipotent adult stem cells with robust in vitro proliferative capacity, which have the ability to differentiate into diverse cell types including those of mesodermal (such as osteogenic, adipogenic, and chondrogenic), endodermal (such as hepatocyte-like cells), and ectodermal (such as neural cells) origin [3, 4]. MSCs can be further characterized by cell membrane antigen expression and their ability to adhere to plastic in vitro [4]. The cell division rate and differentiation capabilities of

Michael S. Pepper and Melvin A. Ambele (eds.), *Adipogenesis: Methods and Protocols*, Methods in Molecular Biology, vol. 2938,
https://doi.org/10.1007/978-1-0716-4607-6_18,

MSCs are inherently determined by their source and can therefore vary widely across donors and tissue types [5, 6]. MSCs secrete signaling molecules that maintain cell survival and growth and regulate inflammatory and immune processes [7, 8]. The potential therapeutic efficacy of MSCs is primarily attributed to these paracrine factors (cytokines and growth factors) [8] and is not derived from engraftment and subsequent differentiation and proliferation of these cells, as engrafted cell longevity has been observed to be transient [9]. MSCs do not express high levels of HLA-I and lack the expression of HLA-II and associated co-stimulatory molecules, which allows them to evade recipient immune responses when utilized in allogeneic transplantation settings. These characteristics position MSCs as promising candidates for clinical application, as evidenced by over 1500 ongoing clinical trials focusing on this cell type registered on ClinicalTrials.gov. A potential future challenge, however, lies in obtaining sufficient quantities of standardized MSCs for therapeutic purposes, as primary isolated MSCs exhibit limitations when considering ex vivo proliferation capacity as well as their characteristic inherent heterogeneity.

Pluripotency can be defined as the ability of a cell to differentiate into cell types from each principal germ layer—ectoderm, mesoderm, and endoderm. Pluripotent cells are naturally found within the inner cell mass of the blastocyst during embryonic development and, in this context, are termed human embryonic stem cells (hESCs). The use of these cells for research purposes has proved to be a strong point of ethical contention, as it would involve the destruction of a human embryo. Induced pluripotent stem cells (iPSCs) are differentiated cells that have been reprogrammed into a pluripotent state [10]. The original observation followed on from the introduction of four transcription factors (*Oct3/4*, *Sox2*, *c-Myc*, and *Klf4*) into fibroblasts, which were reprogramed to become pluripotent [10, 11]. Of significant importance is that these cells have been shown to possess congruent proliferation and differentiation capacities to hESCs. Their use however mitigates any of the aforementioned ethical concerns surrounding embryonic termination. Following on from the initial creation of iPSCs, many researchers have developed iPSC differentiation protocols in order to generate and study cell types of interest. This has alleviated the need for invasive tissue sampling procedures when studying organ-specific cell populations. Moreover, as cell and gene therapy strategies advance, the need for reliable and reproducible cell sources has increased. iPSC-based differentiation strategies present a promising solution to this challenge, as a genetically homogenous iPS cell line can yield an indefinite quantity of desired cell types for therapeutic purposes, thus avoiding the inherent heterogeneity associated with primary cells.

Here, we present a differentiation method used to derive MSC-like cells from iPSCs. The differentiated cells can be characterized to confirm MSC-like attributes as per the established criteria for MSC characterization [12–14].

## 2 Materials

### 2.1 iPSC Culture

1. Human iPSC lines: SC11-010; PCBC03hsi2011080403, SC12-020; PCBC05hsi2012061402, SC14-069; PCBC03hsi2014031101.
2. mTeSR™1 iPSC media.
3. Dulbecco's Modified Eagle Medium/Nutrient Mixture F-12 (DMEM-F12): In a biosafety cabinet, combine 450 mL of DMEM-F12 basal medium, and supplement it with 50 mL of fetal bovine serum (FBS). Mix thoroughly using a sterile 25 mL serological pipette and a pipette controller. Aliquot into 100 mL sterile glass bottles.
4. ROCK (Y-27632) inhibitor stock solution (10 mM): Under sterile cell culture conditions, add 478.1 μL of sterile water to a sterile 2 mL microcentrifuge tube. Add 1 mL of sterile water to a procured tube containing 5 mg of ROCK inhibitor. Mix thoroughly by pipetting up and down, and add it to the 2 mL microcentrifuge. Take up 1 mL of the ROCK inhibitor solution, and add it back to the tube that contained the powder. Perform a wash step to collect any remaining residue, and add the solution back to the microcentrifuge tube. Mix thoroughly using a pipette until dissolved. The stock solution should be divided into aliquots (between 100 and 200 μL) and can be stored at −80 °C for up to a year. Working aliquots can be stored at 4 °C for up to a month.
5. CloneR™2 supplement.
6. CryoStor® CS10.
7. Mr. Frosty™ Freezing Container.
8. Isopropyl alcohol.
9. Sterile 6-well and 96-well plates.
10. 25-, 75-, and 175-$cm^2$ tissue culture flasks.
11. 1.5 and 2 mL microcentrifuge tubes.
12. 15 mL Falcon tubes.
13. Pipettes and sterile tips.
14. Versene.
15. Phosphate-buffered saline (PBS): Dissolve a PBS tablet in 100 mL of distilled water, and mix using a magnetic stirrer. Once fully dissolved, adjust the pH to 7.4.
16. Hemocytometer.

17. hESC-qualified Matrigel/Cultrex/Geltrex: Thaw Matrigel stock [9–11 μg/μL] stored at −80 °C on ice. Make 300 μL aliquots of Matrigel to avoid multiple freeze–thaw cycles using previously cooled tips and tubes. Store 300 μL of Matrigel aliquots at −20 °C until use.

### 2.2 Differentiation Induction

1. Complete Knockout DMEM: Under sterile cell culture conditions, combine 450 mL of Knockout DMEM basal medium, and supplement it with 50 mL of FBS. Mix thoroughly using a sterile 25 mL serological pipette and a pipette controller. Aliquot into 100 mL glass bottles.
2. CD24–phycoerythrin (PE) and CD105–fluorescein isothiocyanate (FITC) antibodies.
3. Gelatinized 10-cm dishes.
4. Accutase.
5. DMEM-F12.
6. Basic fibroblast growth factor (bFGF) stock solution: Under sterile cell culture conditions, add 500 μL of sterile water to the procured tube containing 50 μg of bFGF to achieve a stock solution of 100 μg/mL.
7. Platelet-derived growth factor (PDGF)–AB stock solution: Under sterile cell culture conditions, add 500 μL of sterile water to the procured tube containing 50 μg of PDGF–AB to achieve a stock solution of 100 μg/mL.
8. Epidermal growth factor (EGF) stock solution: Under sterile conditions, add 1 mL of sterile water to the procured tube containing 100 μg of EGF to achieve a stock solution of 100 μg/mL.
9. MSC differentiation and culture medium: In a biosafety cabinet, add 100 mL complete Knockout DMEM to a 100 mL sterile Schott bottle. Add 10 μL of the bFGF, PDGF-AB, and EGF stock solution, to achieve a final concentration of 10 ng/μ L of each cytokine. Mix thoroughly using a 25 mL serological pipette and pipette controller.

### 2.3 Mesenchymal Stromal Cell Characterization

1. Blocking buffer for flow cytometry: To make a 1% bovine serum albumin (BSA) solution, add 1 g of BSA to 100 mL of sterile PBS.
2. Adipocytic differentiation medium: Add 98.546 mL of complete DMEM media to 100 mL glass bottle under sterile conditions. Add 10 μL (1 μM) of the dexamethasone stock solution, 1 ml (10 μg/mL) of the insulin stock solution, 100 μL (0.5 mM) of the 3-isobutyl-1-methylxanthine stock solution, and 354 μL (200 μM) of the indomethacin stock

solution. Mix thoroughly using a 25 mL stripette and pipette controller.

3. Dexamethasone stock solution: 10 mM solution available from suppliers.
4. Insulin stock solution (1 mg/mL): Add 24 mL of sterile 0.005 N HCl (available for purchase) to a sterile 50 mL glass bottle. Add 1 mL of the sterile HCL to the procured bottle containing 25 mg of insulin. Mix thoroughly using a pipette tip. Add the 1 mL to the 24 mL, and mix thoroughly. Perform a number of wash steps using the HCL contained in the glass bottle to fully dissolve the insulin powder. Once fully dissolved, aliquot the stock solution into 1 mL aliquots, and store at − 20 °C.
5. 3-Isobutyl-1-methylxanthine stock solution (500 mM): Add 899 μL of DMSO to a procured tube containing 100 mg of 3-isobutyl-1-methylxanthine. Mix thoroughly with a pipette, until the powder is dissolved. To assist with this, the tube may be gently warmed.
6. Indomethacin stock solution (56.4 mM): Add 48.5 mL of dimethylformamide to a 50 mL glass bottle. Add 1 mL to the procured tube containing 1 g of indomethacin, and mix thoroughly by pipetting up and down. Add the 1 mL to the 48.5 mL and mix thoroughly. Perform a number of wash steps using the dimethylformamide contained in the glass bottle to fully dissolve the powder. Once achieved, store as 360 μL aliquots at −20 °C. Indomethacin is light sensitive; therefore, it is imperative to employ measures that reduce the chance of exposure.
7. Chondrocytic differentiation medium: Add 98.5 mL of complete DMEM media to sterile 100 mL glass bottle. Add 10 μL (0.1 μM) of the dexamethasone working solution, 390 μL (195 μM) ascorbate-2-phosphate, 10 μL (10 ng/mL) transforming growth factor beta 3 (TGF-β3), 35 μL (40 μg/mL) L-proline, 90 μL (100 μg/mL) sodium pyruvate, and 1 mL (1% w/v) ITS+ Universal Culture supplement. Mix thoroughly using a 25 mL stripette and pipette controller.
8. Dexamethasone stock solution: 10 mM solution available from suppliers. Working solution: Add 1 μL of the stock solution to 9 μL of sterile cell culture water to create a solution of 1 mM.
9. Ascorbate-2-phosphate stock solution (50 mM): Add 171 μL of 1 M HCL (available for purchase) to a 1.5 mL tube. Add a further 1 mL to the procured tube containing 15 mg of ascorbate-2-phosphate, and mix thoroughly by pipetting up and down. Add the 1 mL to the 171 μL and mix thoroughly. Perform a number of wash steps using the HCl contained in

the tube to fully dissolve the powder. Once achieved, store as 410 μL aliquots at −20 °C.

10. Transforming growth factor (TGF)-β3 stock solution: Under sterile conditions, add 1 mL of sterile water to the procured tube containing 100 μg of TGF-β3 to achieve a stock solution of 100 μg/mL.
11. Proline stock solution (1 M): Using an analytical balance, weigh off 11.51 g of L-proline powder. Add the powder to a sterile 250 mL Schott bottle, and dissolve in 80 mL of sterile PBS. Once the powder is completely dissolved, add additional PBS to reach a final volume of 100 mL to achieve a stock concentration of 1 M. Ensure complete dissolution by gently warming the solution or using a magnetic stirrer. Filter sterilize the solution using a 0.22 μm filter, under sterile conditions. The stock solution should be stored as 5 mL aliquots at −20 °C to avoid repeated freeze–thaw cycles.
12. Pyruvate stock solution (1 M): Using an analytical balance, weigh off 11 g of sodium pyruvate powder. Add the powder to a sterile 250 mL Schott bottle, and dissolve in 80 mL of sterile cell culture grade water. Once the powder is completely dissolved, add additional cell culture grade water to reach a final volume of 100 mL to achieve a stock concentration of 1 M. Ensure complete dissolution by gently warming the solution or using a magnetic stirrer. Filter sterilize the solution using a 0.22 μm filter, under sterile conditions. The stock solution should be stored as 5 mL aliquots at −20 °C to avoid repeated freeze–thaw cycles.
13. *Osteogenic differentiation medium*: Add 94.5 mL of complete DMEM media to 100 mL glass bottle under sterile conditions. Add 5 mL (10 mM) of β-glycerol phosphate stock solution, 10 μL (0.1 μM) of the dexamethasone working solution, and 500 μL (50 μM) of the ascorbate-2-phosphate stock solution. Mix thoroughly using a 25 mL stripette and pipette controller.
14. β-Glycerol phosphate stock solution: 200 mM solution available from suppliers.
15. Dexamethasone stock solution: 10 mM solution available from suppliers. Working solution: Add 1 μL of the stock solution to 9 μL of sterile cell culture water to create a solution of 1 mM.
16. Ascorbate-2-phosphate stock solution (10 mM): Add 2.9047 mL of 1 M HCL (available for purchase) to a 15 mL tube. Add a further 1 mL to the procured tube containing 10 mg of ascorbate-2-phosphate, and mix thoroughly by pipetting up and down. Add the 1 mL to the 2.9047 mL, and mix thoroughly. Perform a number of wash steps using the HCl contained in the tube to fully dissolve the powder. Once achieved, store as 550 μL aliquots at −20 °C.

17. Sudan Black B stain for adipogenesis: Weigh 500 mg of Sudan Black B, and add it to 20 mL of acetone, followed by 15 mL of acetic acid and 85 mL of water. Stir the solution for 30 min using a magnetic stirrer, and filter it using Whatman paper to remove any remaining particles. Store at room temperature.
18. Sudan Black B destaining solution: Measure 150 mL of acetic acid into a glass beaker, and then add 200 mL of acetone and 650 mL of water.
19. Alizarin Red staining for osteogenesis: Weigh 2 g of Alizarin Red S, and add to 100 mL distilled water in a glass bottle. Adjust the pH to 4.3 using hydrochloric acid or sodium hydroxide, when required. Stir the solution for 30 min using a magnetic stirrer and filter it using Whatman paper to remove any remaining particles. Store at room temperature.
20. Alcian Blue stain for chondrogenesis: Weigh 1 g of Alcian Blue, and add it to 100 mL of 0.1 N HCl (available from suppliers) within a 100 mL glass bottle. Stir the solution for 30 min using a magnetic stirrer, and filter it using Whatman paper to remove any remaining particles. Store at room temperature.

### 2.4 Laboratory Equipment

1. Incubator (37 °C, 5% $CO_2$).
2. Centrifuge.
3. Microscope (inverted fluorescence microscope).
4. EVOS microscope (preferably within BSC).
5. Flow cytometer (for analysis of cell surface markers).
6. Cell sorter.
7. Class II A2 Biosafety Cabinet (BSC).

## 3 Methods

The day-to-day iPSC culture procedures described below have been adapted from a protocol published by Nishihara et al. 2021 [15].

### 3.1 Coating of Cell Culture Plates with Matrigel

1. Thaw a single 300 μL Matrigel aliquot on ice or at 4 °C. Add 30 mL of cold DMEM-F12 (SFM) into a 50 mL Falcon tube. Remove 1 mL, and add it to the Matrigel/Cultrex/Geltrex 300 μL aliquot, and mix thoroughly by pipetting up and down. Add the Matrigel media solution to the 50 mL Falcon tube, and mix using a 25 mL serological pipette. Add 1 mL of this solution to each well in a 6-well plate and 500 μL to each well in a 12-well plate (this is dependent on the number of plates needed for iPS cell culture as well as cells needed for differentiation). Ensure that the entire plate surface is covered by tapping on each side.

2. Incubate the coated plates (37 °C, 5% $CO_2$) for at least 1 h before use (*see* **Note 1**).

### 3.2 Preparation of iPSC Media

A range of well-characterized cell culture media can be used to culture iPSCs. The media selected for your experimental procedures will depend on the media in which the iPSC lines were first seeded as well as the reports/technical data sheets accompanying the cells, provided by researchers or commercial entities. For this protocol, the researchers have selected mTeSR™1 media.

1. Complete mTeSR™1 medium: Thaw mTeSR™1 5× supplement; warm to room temperature, and mix thoroughly by inverting the supplement two to three times. The mTeSR™1 5× supplement may appear slightly cloudy after thawing. If this occurs, place it in a 37 °C water bath for approximately 5 min, swirling occasionally until it becomes clear (*see* **Note 2**).
2. Add 100 mL of mTeSR™1 5× supplement to 400 mL of mTeSR™1 basal medium, and mix thoroughly.

   Aliquot complete mTeSR™1 medium into five 100 mL sterile Schott bottles. Store the bottles in use at 4 °C for up to 2 weeks. If not used immediately, store complete mTeSR™1 medium at −20 °C for up to 6 months. Do not exceed the shelf life of the individual components.

### 3.3 Thawing iPSCs

1. Add 4 mL of pre-warmed mTeSR™1 media into a designated 15 mL Falcon tube, prior to retrieving an iPSC cryovial from liquid nitrogen storage.
2. Retrieve a cryovial, and thaw by applying manual friction (your hands) to the cryovial (*see* **Note 3**).
3. Add 1 mL of pre-warmed mTeSR™1 media to the cryovial. Gently mix the cell suspension with a pipette once and draw up 1 mL. This is to prevent the mechanical disruption of iPSC clumps.
4. Add the 1 mL cell suspension to the 15 mL tube. Draw up 1 mL from this 15 mL tube, and add the cell suspension back to the cryovial to collect any remaining cells. Add the remaining cell suspension to the 15 mL tube, and mix gently using a pipette, but not more than once.
5. Centrifuge the 15 mL tube at 200×*g* for 5 min.
6. Aspirate the supernatant from the 15 mL tube, and resuspend the cell pellet in 2 mL mTeSR™1 media containing ROCK inhibitor (1:2000). Usually, one cryovial (obtained from cryopreserving a single well) is reseeded into two wells (*see* **Note 4**).
7. Remove coating matrix from the 6-well plate in preparation for iPS cell seeding.

8. After adding 1 mL cell suspension and mTeSR™1 media to a final volume of 2 mL, place the plate in an incubator (37 °C, 5% $CO_2$), and move it side to side and back and forth to distribute the cells (DO NOT swirl the plate).
9. Incubate overnight at 37 °C, 5% $CO_2$.

### 3.4 Passaging iPSCs

1. Label a newly coated 6-well plate with the iPSC line name, passage number, date, and your initials.
2. Aspirate Matrigel/Cultrex/Geltrex from the wells you will be using, and add 1 mL of pre-warmed mTeSR™1 media to the two wells.
3. Add 1 mL of mTeSR™1 media to a 15 mL Falcon tube in preparation (when passaging a single well).
4. A well should be passaged once 70–80% confluency is reached. Following a confluency assessment, aspirate mTeSR™1 media from the well you wish to passage.
5. Add 1 mL of Versene and swirl it around the well.
6. Remove Versene once the surface has been coated.
7. To determine the optimum incubation time period, observe the iPSC colonies under a microscope, and once gaps start to develop within highly dense colonies, continue with the following steps.
8. Release 1 mL of mTeSR™1 media with force over the center of the well in order to neutralize the chelating reaction and to remove selected colonies from the well surface (*see* **Note 5**).
9. Take 1 mL of the cell suspension from the well, and add it to the prepared 15 mL tube. Release the cells gently into the media as you do not wish to mechanically disrupt iPSC colonies.
10. Take up 2 mL of cell suspension, and add 1 mL to two wells in the prepared 6-well plate (final volume 2 mL).
11. Place the plate in an incubator, and move it side to side and back and forth to distribute the cells (DO NOT swirl the plate).
12. Incubate overnight at 37 °C, 5% $CO_2$.

### 3.5 Cryopreserving iPSCs

1. Clearly label a single cryovial (for cryopreservation of a single well) with the iPSC line name, passage number, date, and your initials.
2. An iPSC line can be cryopreserved once a 6-well plate has reached 70–80% confluency. Following a confluency assessment, aspirate mTeSR™1 media from the well you wish to passage.
3. Add 1 mL of Versene and swirl it around the well.

4. Remove Versene once the surface has been coated.
5. Incubate the cells at 37 °C, 5% $CO_2$ for the optimized time period.
6. Release 1 mL of CryoStor® CS10 with force over the center of the well to remove selected colonies from the well surface (*see* **Note 5**).
7. Add the cell suspension to the already labelled cryovial, and place it in a Mr. Frosty™ containing isopropyl alcohol. Store in a −80 °C freezer overnight, and transfer to liquid nitrogen storage the following day.

### 3.6 Differentiation Induction

The MSC differentiation protocol described in this chapter has been adapted from the protocols published by Lian et al. 2010 [12] and Nishihara et al. 2021 [15]. This is a 2D differentiation (monolayer) method; however, evidence suggests that iPSC-derived cells obtained from 3D differentiation methods (embryoid body) are more representative of their in vivo counterparts [16]. This area of research is still in its infancy; therefore, further work needs to be performed to fully characterize iPSC-derived MSCs and assess their reliability as an MSC source.

Prior to initiating MSC differentiation, iPSCs, usually passaged and grown as colonies, need to be dissociated into single cells. This is achieved by incubating the iPSCs with the dissociation reagent, Accutase. Differentiation of an iPSC line should occur when at least one well has reached 80–90% confluency.

1. Label a new 12-well plate with the line name, passage number, date, and your initials.
2. Coat each well in a 12-well plate with Matrigel/Cultrex/Geltrex by adding 0.5 mL of the working solution to each well. Ensure the entire surface is covered by tapping the plate on each side (*see* **Note 6**).
3. Incubate the Matrigel-coated plate at 37 °C for at least an hour before use.
4. Add 4 mL of mTeSR™1 media to a labelled 15 mL Falcon tube in preparation for the cell suspension.
5. Aspirate mTeSR™1 media from the well you wish to seed for the differentiation.
6. Add 1 mL of Accutase, and incubate for approximately 7 min at 37 °C to obtain single cells.
7. After the incubation period, use a pipette to gently dislodge any remaining iPSCs attached to the well surface by pipetting up and down three to four times. This will also assist with obtaining a single cell suspension.

8. Add the cell suspension to a prepared 15 mL Falcon tube and mix once or twice.
9. Perform a single wash step using the cell suspension in the Falcon tube to collect any remaining iPSCs in the well. Add it to the 15 mL Falcon tube, and mix gently once to distribute the cells equally.
10. Determine the cell count using a hemocytometer, and calculate the amount of cell suspension required to seed at the required density (5000 cells/cm$^2$) (*see* **Note 7**).
11. Combine mTeSR™1 medium with the cell suspension to achieve the desired seeding density when adding 1 mL to each well.
12. Add ROCK inhibitor (1:2000) to the cell suspension prior to seeding.
13. Remove the Matrigel solution from the wells; you will be using in the labelled 12-well plate and add 1 mL of cell suspension to each well.
14. Distribute the cells around the wells by placing the plate in an incubator and moving it side to side and back and forth. Do not swirl the plate as this will cause the cells to pool at the center of the well.
15. Incubate for 3 days, and change medium every day. Monitor the wells daily for sheets of cells that lift off. If this occurs, it will indicate that the seeding density was too high. This experiment should be aborted and repeated with a lower seeding density.

    The specific concentrations of growth factors and cytokines may vary depending on the iPSC line and the desired differentiation outcome. It is recommended to optimize these conditions through experimentation. Additionally, other factors such as the culture surface and the presence of small molecule inhibitors may also influence differentiation efficiency.
16. After the 3-day incubation period, prepare the differentiation medium as described above (*see* **Note 8**).
17. Aspirate the mTeSR™1 medium, and add 1 mL of the differentiation medium to each well. When adding, place the pipette tip on the side of the well, and release the differentiation medium slowly. This will prevent the attached cells from lifting.
18. Culture the iPSCs with differentiation medium for the optimized duration (typically 14–21 days), and change the media every day.
19. Remove differentiation media from all the wells containing differentiated cells and add 1 mL of Accutase solution to each well.

20. Incubate for 7 min at 37 °C.
21. During this time, place a 40-μm cell strainer into a 50 mL Falcon tube using sterilized forceps (*see* **Note 9**).
22. Add 1 mL of complete DMEM-F12 medium to the cell strainer. Tap the Falcon tube on the side until the surface tension breaks and the 1 mL of media filters through into the Falcon tube.
23. Add the remaining 23 mL (a total of 24 mL for two 12-well plates) of complete DMEM-F12 medium.
24. After the 7 min incubation, detach any remaining cells in the well by pipetting up and down, and add the cell suspension to the strainer. Repeat this step for every well.
25. Once complete, add 1 mL of complete DMEM-F12 medium to each well in the plate to collect any remaining cells. Transfer the collected cells to the cell strainer.
26. Centrifuge the cells at 300×*g* for 10 min, and resuspend in 3 mL of DMEM-F12 medium.
27. Determine the cell count using a hemocytometer, and incubate the cell suspension with the appropriate concentration of CD24-PE and CD105-FITC antibodies.
28. Sort for the CD24-CD105+ cell population using a sterile fluorescent activated cell sorter (FACS) system (*see* **Note 10**).
29. Seed sorted cells in a 6-well plate at 10,000 cells per well, and culture the cells in knockout DMEM supplemented with 10% FBS, bFGF, PDGF-AB, and EGF.
30. When the cells are 70–80% confluent, passage them as previously described and sort one cell into each well of a Matrigel-coated 96-well plate using a cell sorter (*see* **Note 11**). iPSCs do not prefer to grow as single cells; therefore, it may be necessary to add CloneR™2 supplement to the MSC media.
31. Allow them to expand and change media at the end of every week (*see* **Note 12**).
32. Once the single-cell colonies are 80–90% confluent, transfer them to a 12-well plate, and allow them to expand and change media every 2–3 days.
33. Expand the colonies until they reach 70–80% confluency, and then transfer the colonies to a 6-well plate. Allow them to expand and change media every 2–3 days.
34. Once confluent, cryopreserve a proportion of the cells to create cell stocks for long-term use and downstream analysis.

**Table 1**
**Antibodies used to assess MSC markers using flow cytometry**

| | |
|---|---|
| CD14 | CD90 |
| CD11b | HLA-DR |
| CD49d | CD105 |
| CD49b | CD73 |
| CD34 | HLA-ABC |
| CD146 | CD44 |
| CD45 | CD29 |
| CD31 | CD117 |
| CD13 | EpCAM |
| CD24 | NCAM |

### 3.7 Immunophenotypic Characterization of Mesenchymal Stromal Cell

Characterization is an essential component of iPSC research, as it allows one to fully assess the cell types generated through differentiation. Researchers are able to assess cell morphology (*see* **Note 13**), immunophenotype, differentiation potential, and function through the experiments described in detail below. While these methods do provide an overview of the derived cell types, they are not sensitive enough to provide an in-depth analysis. Therefore, it is vital to perform single-cell transcriptomics coupled with relevant functional assays to fully assess these cells, as well as to determine their maturity. Additionally, relevant controls, such as primary MSCs, will need to be obtained to provide a standard to which to compare the iPSC-derived MSCs.

In order to determine if the differentiation was successful, the expression of recognized MSC markers (e.g., CD73, CD90, CD105) and the absence of other markers (e.g., CD34, CD45) can be assessed using flow cytometry (*see* ref. Lian et al. 2007 [17] and Chen et al. 2012 [13]).

1. Passage cells as described above (Subheading 3.6, **steps 5–9**), and determine the cell count using a hemocytometer.
2. Add $2 \times 10^6$ iPSC-derived MSCs to two 1.5 mL tubes; centrifuge at $3500\times g$ for 3 min, and discard the supernatant.
3. Wash the cells once with 1 mL of phosphate-buffered saline (PBS), and incubate with 1 mL of blocking buffer for 30 min to 1 h at room temperature.
4. Dilute the fluorophore-conjugated antibodies (Table 1) as per each manufacturer's recommendations in blocking buffer, and add 50 μL of the solution to $1 \times 10^5$ cells in one tube.

5. Dilute appropriate isotype control antibodies in blocking buffer as per each manufacturer's recommendations, and add 50 μL of the solution to $1 \times 10^5$ cells in a separate tube.
6. Mix and incubate in the dark at room temperature for 15 min.
7. Perform two wash steps with PBS, and then fix the cells by adding 500 μL of 4% paraformaldehyde (PFA), and incubate for 45 min at room temperature.
8. Wash the fixed cells once with PBS and then resuspend them in 500 μL of PBS.
9. Wash unbound antibody, and dye by adding 3 mL of PBS to the cell suspensions and centrifuging for 10 min at 500×*g*.
10. Discard the supernatant and resuspend the cell pellet in 300 μL PBS.
11. Analyze all cell populations using a CytoFLEX flow cytometer.
12. MSC-like cells should be immunophenotyped as being positive for CD73 (ecto-5′-nucleotidase), CD90 (thy-1 membrane glycoprotein), and CD105 (endoglin) and negative for CD34 (hematopoietic progenitor cell marker), CD45 (Pan-hematopoietic marker), and HLA-DR (major histocompatibility complex class II—low expression).

## 4 Notes

1. Plates can be left in the incubator for up to a week, as long as the well surface remains covered with Matrigel solution.
2. Once thawed, use the supplement immediately, or aliquot and store at −20 °C for up to 3 months. Do not exceed the shelf life of the supplement. After thawing the aliquoted supplement, use immediately. Do not refreeze aliquots.
3. Dimethyl sulfoxide (DMSO) is commonly used as a cryoprotectant when freezing cells. After thawing, DMSO should be rapidly diluted by adding culture medium, as prolonged exposure to DMSO can be toxic to cells. DO NOT completely thaw the contents of cryovials; leave a block of ice in the cryovial that will thaw following the addition of the media.
4. Cells are resuspended and plated according to multiple factors—proliferation rate, ability to spontaneously differentiate, etc. This process must be optimized according to each iPSC line.
5. iPSC colonies at the center of the well are usually undifferentiated, with differentiated colonies present around the perimeter. This is not always the case; therefore, it is vital to monitor your lines daily and select the area of the well you wish to passage.

The presence of differentiated colonies will reduce the efficiency of your differentiation protocol, as spontaneously differentiated cells appear to be of a neuronal nature, and will be resistant to any further differentiation.

6. At least six wells should be seeded for one iPSC line to ensure a sufficient number of differentiated cells for further experimentation and downstream analysis.
7. As part of your initial differentiation experiments, test a range of seeding densities (75,000–400,000 cells/well) to determine the optimal density for future use. Note that this may vary between different iPSC lines.
8. The differentiation medium should be freshly prepared every week; therefore, only prepare enough medium for 1 week at a time. Store at 4 °C.
9. Take care not to damage the filter in the process, as clumps of cells in the cell suspension may hinder the sorting process.
10. If a FACS system is not available, sorting for CD105+ cells can be performed using magnetic-activated cell sorting (MACS); however, the CD24− cell population cannot be removed during this initial step. A second MACS step could be added after expanding the CD105+ population to collect the flow-through (CD24− population).
11. If a sorter is not available, single cells can be isolated using limiting dilutions.
12. It may be difficult to see the single-cell clones initially. However, allow them to expand for up to a month. Monitor the plates weekly, and exclude wells that have more than one cell colony.
13. iPSC-derived MSCs should be observed under a light microscope for the characteristic spindle-shaped MSC morphology. Adherence to plastic should also be assessed.

## Acknowledgements

We would like to thank Dr. Miwako Fujisawa and Prof. Britta Engelhardt at the Theodor Kocher Institute at the University of Bern for their assistance with training in iPSC culture and differentiation. This work was supported by the South African Medical Research Council (Extramural Unit for Stem Cell Research and Therapy) and the University of Pretoria via the Institute for Cellular and Molecular Medicine.

## References


1. Rigotti G, Marchi A, Sbarbati A (2009) Adipose-derived mesenchymal stem cells: past, present, and future. Aesth Plast Surg 33(3): 271–273. https://doi.org/10.1007/s00266-009-9339-7
2. Crisan M et al (2008) A perivascular origin for mesenchymal stem cells in multiple human organs. Cell Stem Cell 3(3):301–313. https://doi.org/10.1016/j.stem.2008.07.003
3. Bieback K, Brinkmann I (2010) Mesenchymal stromal cells from human perinatal tissues: from biology to cell therapy. World J Stem Cells 2(4):81–92. https://doi.org/10.4252/wjsc.v2.i4.81
4. Dominici M et al (2006) Minimal criteria for defining multipotent mesenchymal stromal cells. The International Society for Cellular Therapy position statement. Cytotherapy 8(4):315–317. https://doi.org/10.1080/14653240600855905
5. Barberini DJ et al (2014) Equine mesenchymal stem cells from bone marrow, adipose tissue and umbilical cord: immunophenotypic characterization and differentiation potential. Stem Cell Res Ther 5(1):25. https://doi.org/10.1186/scrt414
6. Xu L et al (2017) Tissue source determines the differentiation potentials of mesenchymal stem cells: a comparative study of human mesenchymal stem cells from bone marrow and adipose tissue. Stem Cell Res Ther 8(1):275. https://doi.org/10.1186/s13287-017-0716-x
7. Sensebe L, Bourin P (2009) Mesenchymal stem cells for therapeutic purposes. Transplantation 87(9 Suppl):S49–S53. https://doi.org/10.1097/TP.0b013e3181a28635
8. Barrachina L et al (2016) Effect of inflammatory environment on equine bone marrow derived mesenchymal stem cells immunogenicity and immunomodulatory properties. Vet Immunol Immunopathol 171:57–65. https://doi.org/10.1016/j.vetimm.2016.02.007
9. Kean TJ, Lin P, Caplan AI, Dennis JE (2013) MSCs: delivery routes and engraftment, cell-targeting strategies, and immune modulation. Stem Cells Int 2013:732742. https://doi.org/10.1155/2013/732742
10. Takahashi K, Yamanaka S (2006) Induction of pluripotent stem cells from mouse embryonic and adult fibroblast cultures by defined factors. Cell 126(4):663–676. https://doi.org/10.1016/j.cell.2006.07.024
11. Takahashi K et al (2007) Induction of pluripotent stem cells from adult human fibroblasts by defined factors. Cell 131(5):861–872. https://doi.org/10.1016/j.cell.2007.11.019
12. Lian Q et al (2010) Functional mesenchymal stem cells derived from human induced pluripotent stem cells attenuate limb ischemia in mice. Circulation 121(9):1113–1123. https://doi.org/10.1161/CIRCULATIONAHA.109.898312
13. Chen YS, Pelekanos RA, Ellis RL, Horne R, Wolvetang EJ, Fisk NM (2012) Small molecule mesengenic induction of human induced pluripotent stem cells to generate mesenchymal stem/stromal cells. Stem Cells Transl Med 1(2):83–95. https://doi.org/10.5966/sctm.2011-0022
14. Luzzani C et al (2015) A therapy-grade protocol for differentiation of pluripotent stem cells into mesenchymal stem cells using platelet lysate as supplement. Stem Cell Res Ther 6(1):6. https://doi.org/10.1186/scrt540
15. Nishihara H, Gastfriend BD, Kasap P, Palecek SP, Shusta EV, Engelhardt B (2021) Differentiation of human pluripotent stem cells to brain microvascular endothelial cell-like cells suitable to study immune cell interactions. STAR Protoc 2(2):100563. https://doi.org/10.1016/j.xpro.2021.100563
16. Majid QA et al (2024) Generation and characterisation of scalable and stable human pluripotent stem cell-derived microvascular-like endothelial cells for cardiac applications. Angiogenesis. https://doi.org/10.1007/s10456-024-09929-5
17. Lian Q et al (2007) Derivation of clinically compliant MSCs from CD105+, CD24− differentiated human ESCs. Stem Cells 25(2): 425–436. https://doi.org/10.1634/stemcells.2006-0420

# Chapter 19

# Isolation and Characterization of Equine Mesenchymal Stromal/Stem Cells

**Lisa Marie Bosman, Melvin A. Ambele, and Michael S. Pepper**

## Abstract

Regenerative medicine is a relatively new branch of therapeutics in equine medicine, which aims to restore and reconstitute tissue function and structure via cellular and/or noncellular approaches. Biological constituents such as mesenchymal stromal/stem cells (MSCs) are potent therapeutics, which can aid in damaged tissue regeneration due to their differentiation capacity into many different cell types such as adipose tissue, bone, and cartilage. MSCs can be successfully and conveniently isolated from equine subcutaneous adipose tissue (adipose-derived stromal cells, ASCs). In horses, there are currently no standardized methods for characterizing ASCs both in research and clinical practice. However, many studies are investigating antibodies which may be expressed on the ASC cell surface through multicolor immunophenotyping. This chapter describes techniques used to isolate, grow, characterize, and store equine ASCs, which have been adapted from extensive published research from the Institute of Cellular and Molecular Medicine (ICMM) at the University of Pretoria.

**Key words** Mesenchymal stromal cells, Adipose tissue, Equine, Regenerative medicine, Cell therapy

## 1 Introduction

Multipotent mesenchymal stromal/stem cells (MSCs) may be useful orthobiologics in horses, due to their proliferation and differentiation capacity into cells such as chondroblasts, osteoblasts, and myoblasts [1], and they can be easily isolated from a variety of sources including adipose tissue (AT), Wharton's jelly (umbilical cord), epidermis, dental pulp, bone marrow, and the placenta [2, 3]. In horses, subcutaneous AT (Sc-AT) is the most common AT to be utilized for adipose-derived stromal/stem cell (ASC) isolation, as it is more accessible than umbilical cord and bone marrow [4]. This chapter describes the isolation of equine ASCs from Sc-AT.

According to the International Federation for Adipose Tissue Therapeutics and Science (IFATS) and the International Society for Cellular Therapy (ISCT), human MSCs are required to fulfil certain

Michael S. Pepper and Melvin A. Ambele (eds.), *Adipogenesis: Methods and Protocols*, Methods in Molecular Biology, vol. 2938, https://doi.org/10.1007/978-1-0716-4607-6_19,

criteria. These include plastic adherence within 24–48 h and the ability to express certain markers with increasing homogeneity through each passage cycle. However, there are no specific internationally accepted standards for equine ASCs as there are for humans. Nonetheless, multiple studies have shown that equine ASCs express CD29, CD44, and CD90 and do not express CD34 and CD45 [5–10]. The methodology presented in part II of this chapter describes the determination of equine ASC cell number and viability and immunophenotypic characterization. The methodology was adapted from published methodology used for human ASCs at the Institute for Cellular and Molecular Medicine [11–21] (*see* Chapter 15).

## 2 Materials

Unless otherwise stated, or during flow cytometry analysis, all procedures and methodologies are conducted in a laminar flow hood under sterile conditions at room temperature (<25 °C). All tubes or flasks containing cells, as well as other reagents, must be closed in the laminar flow hood, prior to their removal from the working sterile conditions and placement into other environments such as an incubator (37 °C at 5% $CO_2$) or refrigerator (~4 °C). The following sections all require the use of a laminar flow hood, 37 °C/5% $CO_2$ incubator, and 37 °C hot box/incubator/water bath, and a large proportion of the methodology requires the use of a centrifuge, light microscope, and flow cytometer. In order to store the isolated stromal vascular fraction (SVF) and/or characterized ASCs, ensure you have access to a −80 °C freezer and liquid nitrogen storage tank/dewar, as viable ASCs cannot be stored in a standard freezer at ~ −20 °C (*see* **Note 1**). This methodology is specific to ASCs grown in T75 flasks, which is what we recommend; however, T25 flasks and 6-well plates can also be used with differing volumes of complete growth medium and PBS for washing. General instructions for both the isolation and characterization of equine ASCs can be seen in **Notes 2–8**.

### 2.1 Isolation

1. Complete Growth Medium (CGM*): Remove approximately 60 mL of Gibco™ Dulbecco's Modified Eagle Medium (DMEM), high glucose, GlutaMAX™ supplement from the 500 mL bottle, and store at −4 °C. To the remaining 440 mL in the bottle, add 10 mL penicillin–streptomycin (Pen/Strep) and 50 mL fetal bovine serum (FBS) to make a 2% Pen/Strep, 10% FBS CGM (*see* **Note 9**). Store the CGM at approximately 4–8 °C until when needed.
2. Phosphate-buffered saline (PBS) containing 2% Pen/Strep: Add 10 mL Pen/Strep to 490 mL PBS (*see* **Note 10**).

3. Surgical blade and holder.
4. Forceps.
5. Tissue culture dish: minimum size of 150 mm.
6. Bottletop filter or syringe filter: 0.22 μM.
7. Collagenase type 1 (0.1%): Weigh 0.1 g collagenase type I powder, and add to 100 mL PBS containing 2% Pen/Strep (*see* **Notes 11–13**) in a Schott bottle. Vortex the solution to ensure complete dissolution. Filter the collagenase solution into a new Schott bottle using the 0.22 μM bottletop filter or syringe filter under sterile conditions in a laminar flow hood.
8. Rotating incubator at 37 °C.
9. Cell strainer: 70 μM.
10. Red blood cell lysing solution (*see* **Note 14**).
11. Fluorescence microscope.
12. Centrifuge.
13. Cell culture flask.
14. Sterile Pasteur pipettes.

### 2.2 Characterization

1. Complete Growth Medium* (CGM) containing 2% Pen/-Strep, 10% FBS CGM (*see* **Note 9**).
2. Phosphate-buffered saline (PBS) containing 2% Pen/Strep.
3. Flow cytometry counting beads or fluorophores. Store at approximately 4–6 °C.
4. Flow cytometry quality control (QC) beads. Store at approximately 4–6 °C.
5. Vybrant™ DyeCycle™ (VDC) Ruby stain (2.5 mM in DMSO). Store at approximately −20 °C, desiccated and protected from light.
6. Equine-specific multicolor antibodies: CD29, CD44, CD90, CD34, and CD45, with each antibody labelled with a different wavelength color marker, to make up a full panel. Store for short-term use in 4–6 °C and for long-term storage −20 °C.

## 3 Methods

Isolation can either be from solid adipose tissue (with or without skin) or liquid lipoaspirate. Pre-warm both the CGM and PBS (2% Pen/Strep) for a minimum of 30 min in a 37 °C hot box, prior to use in order to protect the cells from potential cold shock. Although the characterization procedure uses a flow cytometer in non-sterile conditions, all tube preparation (Subheading 3.2, **step 4**) and cell handling should be completed under sterile conditions in a laminar flow hood.

### 3.1 Isolation

1. *If there is skin present on a solid adipose tissue sample:* With the use of sterile surgical blades and holder, cut a maximum of 75-mm-diameter-sized piece of the full adipose tissue off the skin, and place it in the Petri dish (*see* **Note 15**).
2. *If there is no skin present, or the skin has been removed:* Use the sterile surgical blade, holder, and forceps to mince the tissue into as small as possible pieces (*see* **Note 16**), and place the minced tissue into a 50 mL Falcon tube (Fig. 1).
3. Repeat the procedure, until you have 25 mL of minced tissue per 50 mL Falcon tube (if possible).
4. *For lipoaspirate (liquid):* Distribute 25 mL of lipoaspirate per 50 mL Falcon tube (*see* **Notes 17** and **18**).
5. In each 50 mL centrifuge tube (containing 25 mL of minced adipose tissue), add 25 mL of PBS (2% Pen/Strep) to wash the sample (Fig. 1).
6. Centrifuge the tubes at 1700×*g*, for 3 min (*see* **Note 19**) (Fig. 2).
7. Remove the oily layer on top using an aspirator or sterile Pasteur pipette, and transfer the adipose tissue/lipoaspirate layer into a new 50 mL Falcon tube (*see* **Note 20**), leaving behind the PBS/supernatant. The PBS/supernatant left in the tube can be discarded.
8. Depending on the amount of blood contamination seen in the adipose tissue sample, repeat the washing steps (**steps 5-7**) one or two more times (Fig. 3).

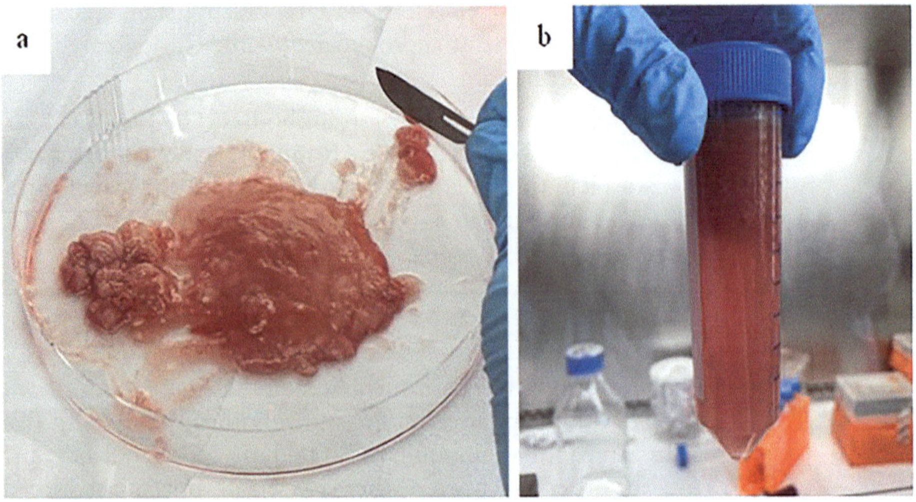


**Fig. 1** Adipose tissue sample in both whole pieces (left) and minced pieces (right) in a 150 mm Petri dish (**a**). The minced adipose tissue is placed into a 50 mL Falcon tube, and PBS (2% Pen/Strep) is then added to the sample (**b**)

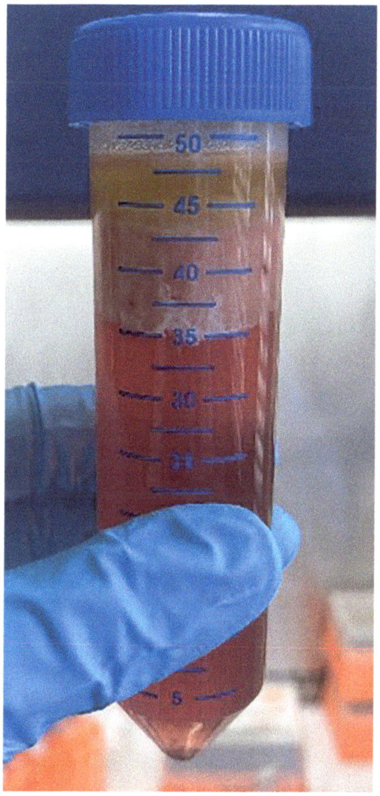

**Fig. 2** After centrifugation, an oil layer can be seen on top of the adipose tissue, followed by a layer of PBS (2% Pen/Strep), and a cell debris pellet at the bottom of the tube

9. Place the tube containing the adipose tissue sample, lid facing down, on an analytical balance, and record the mass in grams. Use a tissue culture dish to keep the balance clean (*see* **Note 21**).
10. Record the volume of adipose tissue inside the 50 mL Falcon tube.
11. Depending on the *volume* recorded in **step 10**, add the same volume of collagenase type I (0.1%) solution into each 50 mL Falcon tube, and incubate the samples for about 45–60 min at 37 °C in a rotating incubator at medium speed (Fig. 4).
12. Centrifuge the tubes for 5 min at 800×*g*, and shake the tube vigorously to disrupt the pellet.
13. Repeat the centrifugation step for 5 min at 800×*g* to separate the sample into its various components (Fig. 5).
14. Remove and discard the digested adipose tissue at the top of the tube using a sterile glass or Pasteur pipette. Once the adipose tissue has been removed, start slowly removing and discarding the collagenase solution, and stop when the total volume is 15 mL (*see* **Note 22**).

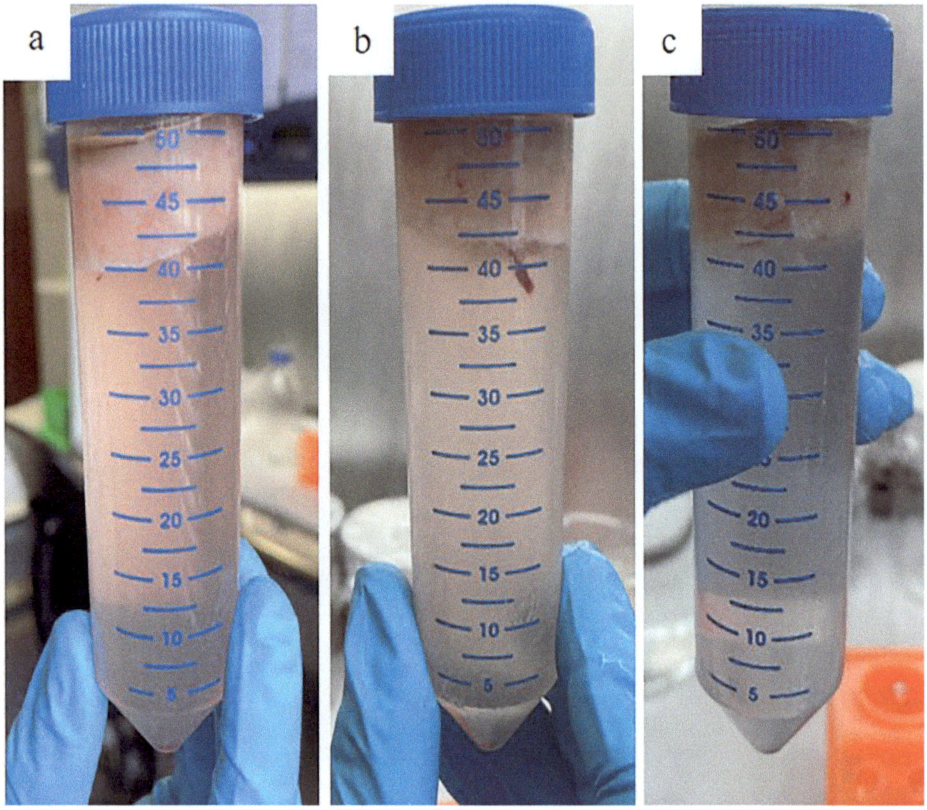

**Fig. 3** Through consecutive washes and centrifugation with PBS (2% Pen/Strep) (**a**–**c**), any blood contamination is removed from the adipose tissue

15. Once again, shake the pellet to resuspend cells in solution, and then filter it through a 70 μM cell strainer into a new 50 mL Falcon tube, to remove undigested tissues and debris (*see* **Note 23**).
16. Centrifuge the tubes with the flow through containing cells in suspension for 5 min at 800×*g*, and then carefully aspirate all the liquid leaving behind the cell pellet.
17. Add 5 mL of CGM to each cell pellet in order to neutralize the collagenase solution. Gently pipette cells in and out to resuspend them in solution, and then combine resuspended cells in a singular tube (if more than one 50 mL Falcon tube of adipose tissue was used).
18. Using PBS, top up the singular tube to 50 mL, and centrifuge at 300×*g* for 5 min. Remove and discard the supernatant without disturbing the cell pellet.
19. Gently resuspend the pellet in approximately 20 mL of red blood cell lysing solution, and incubate for 10 min at room temperature (*see* **Note 24**).

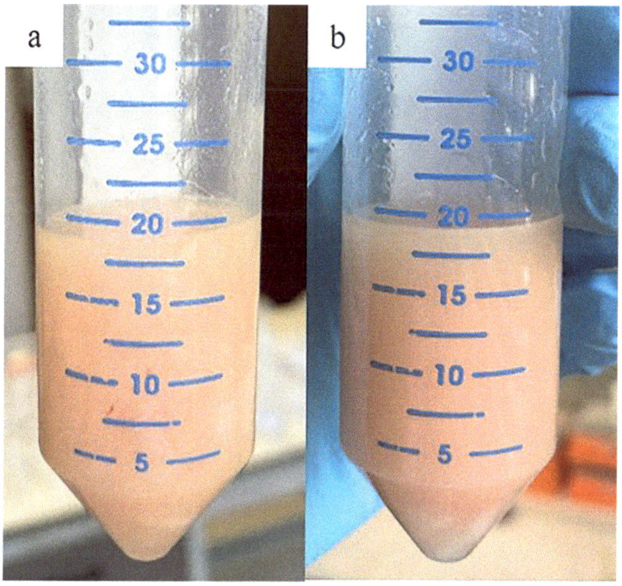


**Fig. 4** The adipose tissue (**a**) is digested with collagenase type I (0.1%) through a 1 h rotating incubation period at 37 °C, to produce a more uniform liquid sample (**b**)

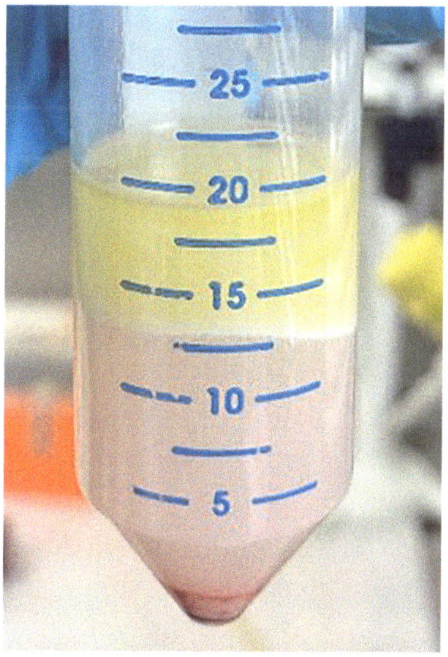

**Fig. 5** After centrifugation, the sample is separated into three clear layers, including an oil and digested adipose tissue layer on top, a collagenase type I (0.1%) solution layer in the middle, and a cellular layer at the bottom

20. Add 20 mL of PBS to the tube to neutralize the lysing solution, and centrifuge at 300×*g* for 5 min.
21. Remove and discard the supernatant from the pellet, and wash the cells by adding 20 mL of PBS solution, and centrifuge for 5 min at 300×*g* (*see* **Note 25**).
22. Remove and discard the supernatant, and resuspend the pellet in approximately 20 mL of CGM.
23. Filter the cells through a 70 μM cell strainer into a new tube.

### 3.2 Characterization

1. Perform the startup procedure of your flow cytometer.
2. Conduct a flow cytometer clean using flow cytometric specific cleaning product and perform a quality control (QC) check using flow cytometry QC beads.
3. Pipette mix the cell suspension to be tested.
4. Set up three separate flow cytometry tubes *per sample* in a laminar flow hood as follows, with specific instructions for each tube. **Tube 1—Unstained** should contain 100 μL cell suspension and 200 μL PBS (2% Pen/Strep). **Tube 2—Count and viability,** should comprise of 100 μL cell suspension, 2 μL of VDC Ruby stain, 100 μL cell counting beads or fluorophores, and 200 μL PBS (2% Pen/Strep). This tube should be incubated in the dark, at room temperature, for 10 min. **Tube 3—Characterization** (*see* **Notes 26–28**) should include 100 μL cell suspension, 200 μL PBS (2% Pen/Strep), and 5 μL of each equine-specific antibody (CD29, CD44, CD90, CD34, and CD45). Tube 3 should be incubated in the dark, at room temperature, for 20 min.
5. Place the **unstained tube (tube 1)** on the flow cytometer pedestal, and run the program (*see* **Note 29**). Gate your sample for autofluorescence and cell populations.
6. Repeat the run **on tube 1** three times to ensure your results are repeatable and validated.
7. Rinse or quick wash the flow cytometer with distilled water, or according to manufacturer's instructions, and discard the flow cytometric tube.
8. Place **tube 2**, the count and viability flow cytometric tube, on the pedestal and run the program. Record the number of cells per microliter, volume of the sample, and viability (% alive).
9. Repeat the run **on tube 2** three times to ensure your results are repeatable and validated.
10. Rinse or quick wash the flow cytometer with distilled water, or according to manufacturer's instructions, and discard the flow cytometric tube.
11. Place **tube 3**, the characterization/immunophenotyping flow cytometric tube, on the pedestal, and run the program. The

cells should have the following antibody expression ($^{+}$) (or lack thereof ($^{-}$)): CD29$^{+}$, CD44$^{+}$, CD90$^{+}$, CD34$^{-}$, and CD45$^{-}$.

12. Repeat the run **on tube 3** three times to ensure your results are repeatable and validated.
13. Rinse or quick wash the flow cytometer with distilled water, or according to manufacturer's instructions, and discard the flow cytometric tube.
14. Proceed with the flow cytometric shutdown procedure according to manufacturer's instructions.
15. In a laminar flow hood, plate the cells at 50,000 nucleated cells/cm$^2$ in T75 flasks according to the tube 2 (count and viability) results captured, with pre-warmed CGM to a maximum of 8 mL. If there are less than 50,000 nucleated cells/cm$^2$, plate in either a T25 flask (maximum of 4 mL CGM and cell solution per flask) or 6-well plate (maximum of 2 mL CGM and cell solution per well) to ensure survivability of the cells (*see* **Note 30**).
16. Label the flasks/plates P0F0, and incubate the cells at 37 °C, 5% $CO_2$ (*see* **Note 31**).
17. At both 24 h, and 48 h, post-seeding, check the flasks/plates for plastic adherence using a light microscope. The cells should not move with the solution if they have adhered to the flasks/plates.
18. 72-hour post-seeding, gently remove and discard the old CGM through aspiration, or by using a sterile Pasteur pipette from each flask/plate (*see* **Note 32**).
19. Add 8 mL PBS (2% Pen/Strep) (T75), 4 mL PBS (2% Pen/-Strep) (T25), or 2 mL PBS (2% Pen/Strep) (6-well plate) to the flasks/plates, and gently swirl the solution to remove non-adherent cells from the flask/plate. Remove and discard the PBS solution through aspiration or via the use of sterile Pasteur pipettes.
20. Feed cells in the flasks/plates by adding 8 mL of CGM (T75), 4 mL CGM (T25), or 2 mL CGM (6-well plate), and place the flasks/plates back in the 37 °C and 5% $CO_2$ incubator.
21. The adherent cells are the MSCs.

## 4 Notes

1. ASCs should be stored at −80 °C overnight, prior to their movement into liquid nitrogen (−196 °C) for long-term storage. This is to prevent cellular damage during freezing, such as the formation of ice crystals at −20 °C which can irreversibly

damage cellular membranes, and to maintain cellular viability and integrity. Additionally, the predominant cryoprotectant used to store ASCs, dimethyl sulfoxide (DMSO), requires extremely low temperatures due to its cytotoxicity effects at temperatures warmer than −196 °C.

2. It is important to note that the use of the cells isolated and characterized in this methodology is *for research purposes only* due to the xenogeneic nature of the fetal bovine serum used as a complete medium supplement. In order to use the ASCs in a clinical setting, the cell culture methodology must be completed according to strict good manufacturing practice (GMP) guidelines in order to ensure quality assurance and quality standards are met, and therefore equine-derived medium additives should be used.
3. MSC quality is highly dependent on the age of the donor and the tissue of origin [22]. For example, human MSCs from younger donors have longer lifespans, increased expansion, improved differentiation, and reduced immunogenicity when compared to older donors [23, 24]. In equine studies, Burk et al. [25] found MSCs derived from Wharton's jelly, tendon, or adipose tissue to give over 200 times higher numbers of cells, than MSCs derived from cord blood or bone marrow.
4. Ensure all experimentation is completed in triplicate with regard to the number of samples and repeats conducted in order to ensure repeatability and validity.
5. Make sure you follow strict instructions on use of a laminar flow hood initiation and shutdown procedures.
6. Use industrial grade ethanol (>99%) or industrial methylated spirits (IMS, >99%) to clean the laminar flow hood, all equipment in the laminar flow hood and anything going into the laminar flow hood prior to immediate use. Please use laboratory best practice guidelines.
7. Check if there is water in incubators, and that it is not contaminated prior to use.
8. Use a non-wipe marker for labelling tubes. The marker notation should not be rubbed off when it comes into contact with ethanol or IMS. If you cannot get a hold of these markers, please use a label making machine to label the tubes and flasks.
9. The concentration of FBS can be increased to 20%, if necessary, yet we find a 10% solution to be more than adequate.
10. We suggest using PBS throughout the methodology; however, Hank's balanced salt solution (HBSS) is recommended by other laboratories.

11. Certain collagenase manufacturers recommend using HBSS to make up the collagenase type I solution. It can be used if preferred and/or if PBS is not available.
12. This should be made fresh for each isolation procedure, and the volume of 0.1% collagenase type I solution made should be the same volume of the adipose tissue isolated after the washing procedure.
13. Add the collagenase type I powder to a Schott bottle, and add the required amount of PBS with 2% Pen/strep, and mix well. For an isolation of 8 × 25 mL, you will need 200 mL of PBS solution.
14. We recommend using the VersaLyse™ Lysing Solution, 1 mL per test. Store at room temperature. This is used to lyse any red blood cells in the sample and prepare the sample for flow cytometry analysis.
15. Do not cut too close to the skin when removing the adipose tissue. This will ensure you do not contaminate the sample with hair follicle or epithelial cells.
16. The more you mince the tissue into smaller pieces, the easier and more complete the enzymatic digestion with collagenase will be. This is due to the increased surface area of the adipose tissue.
17. Try to obtain as much minced tissue as possible to improve on the isolation yield. This will be dependent on what area you have isolated the ASCs from; for example, adipose tissue from the gluteal region can give you a maximum of 100 mL fat. However, up to a total of 16 Falcon tubes (50 mL) of minced fat tissue, or 400 mL of sample, can be gained from abdominal region adipose tissue.
18. Once you have distributed the lipoaspirate into 50 mL centrifuge tubes, let the sample settle. This will allow the lipoaspirate to rise to the top, above the PBS. Only move the lipoaspirate section of the separated sample into the tubes, and not the Ringer's lactate portion. If the sample is runny, fill 16 tubes with the sample, and do an initial spin (3 min at 1700×*g*) before adding PBS to start the wash procedure. This is to separate the tissue from any other liquid present in the sample. After this spin, move 25 mL of sample into the 50 mL tubes, and continue with the washes in **step 2** of the methodology. 16 tubes are used in our methodology only because our centrifuge can hold 16 × 50 mL tubes at a time.
19. After centrifugation, the sample separates into three layers: the bottom layer is PBS/supernatant; the middle layer is the adipose tissue, and the top layer is the oil from the ruptured adipose cells.

20. When transferring the adipose tissue to a new tube, hold the 50 mL tube at a 45° angle, and use a glass pipette or sterile Pasteur pipette to create an air channel (to break the vacuum) at the top of the tube. Slowly pour the compacted adipose tissue into a new 50 mL tube.
21. Wipe down the tubes with paper towel and ethanol, as the oil tends to get everywhere.
22. *Be careful* when removing the digested adipose tissue! Prior to digestion, the ASCs are found in between the adipose tissue; therefore, as you have now digested the tissue, the MSCs have been pelleted through centrifugation at the bottom of the tube, while the collagenase and digested adipose tissue are at the top. Consequently, it is very easy to remove and discard the pellet during this step.
23. The cell strainer can easily become clogged, thereby making filtering difficult. To work around this issue, move a sterile Pasteur pipette up and down to aid in the filtration process. Additionally, you can set up multiple tubes with strainers to let gravity aid you in the filtration process.
24. The lysing solution is used to lyse the remaining red blood cells. This causes the cell pellet to have a reddish color.
25. If the lysing solution has adequately lysed the red blood cells in the pellet, and you have conducted a singular wash with PBS, the pellet should have a creamy white color. If the pellet is still a reddish color at this stage, repeat the lysing (**steps 16–18**), until the solution is a creamy white color.
26. Equine ASCs do not have the same immunophenotyping profile as human ASCs; therefore, it is crucial to confirm with your supplier that your equine-specific antibodies have been validated using equine cells, prior to purchasing them.
27. Ensure your antibodies are labelled with different wave-length markers; otherwise, you will not be able to distinguish between them on a multicolor immunophenotyping panel.
28. Ensure you have tested the antibodies with known and previously characterized equine ASCs, and gated the specific antibodies, on the flow cytometer you plan to use. This will allow you to have controls available and standards to compare your results to.
29. Prior to testing samples using this methodology, please make sure you have a standardized and/or validated gating procedure for ASCs on the flow cytometer for different tests you may be conducting, such as counting, immunophenotyping, proliferation, and viability for ASCs.
30. Use the following calculation to ensure the correct volume of cell suspension is seeded at 50,000 cells/cm$^2$ per flask or well.

The cell count (cells/μL) is the number at the bottom of the equation, and the cell solution (μL) is the volume of cell suspension to add to each flask/well:

$$\textbf{T75 flask}: \frac{3{,}750{,}000\ \text{cells/flask}}{\text{Cells}/\mu\text{L}} = \text{Cell solution } (\mu\text{L}) + 8\ \text{mL CGM}$$

$$\textbf{T25 flask}: \frac{1{,}250{,}000\ \text{cells/flask}}{\text{Cells}/\mu\text{L}} = \text{Cell solution } (\mu\text{L}) + 4\ \text{mL CGM}$$

$$\textbf{Individual wells(6 - well plate)}: \frac{480{,}000\ \text{cells}/\mathit{well}}{\text{Cells}/\mu\text{L}} = \text{Cell solution } (\mu\text{L}) + 2\ \text{mL CGM}$$

31. The cultures should be named according to the specific laboratory naming convention and should start off as **P0F0**, which stands for passage number 0 (as no Trypsin has been used on these cells) and freezing number 0 (as the cells have never been frozen). All data collected on the stromal vascular fraction (SVF) should be labelled as *Culture name_SVF*.
32. Tilt the flask at a 45° angle to remove the old CGM. Do not place the aspirator or sterile Pasteur pipette on the surface where the cells have been cultured to avoid removing healthy cells. Rather place the aspirator glass tip, or sterile Pasteur pipette in the corner of the flaks within the liquid which needs to be removed. Only once all the liquid has been removed, then continue the washing procedure with PBS.

## Acknowledgement

We would like to acknowledge researchers at the Institute for Cellular and Molecular Medicine for their help and previous research methodology in adipose-derived stromal cell procedures. We would also like to acknowledge the team at the Equine Research Centre at the University of Pretoria.

## References

1. Cequier A, Sanz C, Rodellar C, Barrachina L (2021) The usefulness of mesenchymal stem cells beyond the musculoskeletal system in horses. Animals 11(4):931. https://doi.org/10.3390/ani11040931
2. Bunnell BA, Flaat M, Gagliardi C, Patel B, Ripoll C (2008) Adipose-derived stem cells: isolation, expansion and differentiation. Methods (San Diego, Calif) 45(2):115–120. https://doi.org/10.1016/j.ymeth.2008.03.006
3. Zuk PA, Zhu M, Ashjian P, De Ugarte DA, Huang JI, Mizuno H, Alfonso ZC, Fraser JK, Benhaim P, Hedrick MH (2002) Human

adipose tissue is a source of multipotent stem cells. Mol Biol Cell 13(12):4279–4295. https://doi.org/10.1091/mbc.e02-02-0105

4. Trachsel DS, Stage HJ, Rausch S, Trappe S, Söllig K, Sponder G, Merle R et al (2022) Comparison of sources and methods for the isolation of equine adipose tissue-derived stromal/stem cells and preliminary results on their reaction to incubation with 5-azacytidine. Animals 12(16):2049. Retrieved from https://doi.org/10.3390/ani12162049
5. De Schauwer C, Van de Walle GR, Van Soom A, Meyer E (2013) Mesenchymal stem cell therapy in horses: useful beyond orthopedic injuries? Vet Q 33(4):234–241. https://doi.org/10.1080/01652176.2013.800250
6. Ranera B, Lyahyai J, Romero A, Vázquez FJ, Remacha AR, Bernal ML, Zaragoza P, Rodellar C, Martín-Burriel I (2011) Immunophenotype and gene expression profiles of cell surface markers of mesenchymal stem cells derived from equine bone marrow and adipose tissue. Vet Immunol Immunopathol 144(1–2): 147–154. https://doi.org/10.1016/j.vetimm.2011.06.033
7. Barberini DJ, Freitas NPP, Magnoni MS et al (2014) Equine mesenchymal stem cells from bone marrow, adipose tissue and umbilical cord: immunophenotypic characterization and differentiation potential. Stem Cell Res Ther 5(25):1–11. https://doi.org/10.1186/scrt414
8. Paebst F, Piehler D, Brehm W, Heller S, Schroeck C, Tárnok A, Burk J (2014) Comparative immunophenotyping of equine multipotent mesenchymal stromal cells: an approach toward a standardized definition. Cytometry A 85(8):678–687. https://doi.org/10.1002/cyto.a.22491
9. Hillmann A, Ahrberg AB, Brehm W, Heller S, Josten C, Paebst F, Burk J (2016) Comparative characterization of human and equine mesenchymal stromal cells: a basis for translational studies in the equine model. Cell Transplant 25(1):109–124. https://doi.org/10.3727/096368915X687822
10. Arnhold S, Elashry MI, Klymiuk MC, Geburek F (2019) Investigation of stemness and multipotency of equine adipose-derived mesenchymal stem cells (ASCs) from different fat sources in comparison with lipoma. Stem Cell Res Ther 10(1):309. https://doi.org/10.1186/s13287-019-1429-0
11. Durandt C, Pepper MS (2016) Isolation and characterization of adipose-derived stromal cells. In: Stem cells in clinical applications. Springer, pp 131–161. https://doi.org/10.1007/978-3-319-40073-0
12. van Vollenstee FA, Hoffmann D, Pepper MS (2016) Harvesting and collection of adipose tissue for the isolation of adipose-derived stromal/stem cells. In: Stem cells in clinical applications. Springer, pp 199–220. https://doi.org/10.1007/978-3-319-40073-0
13. Ambele MA, Dessels C, Durandt C, Pepper MS (2016) Genome-wide analysis of gene expression during adipogenesis in human adipose-derived stromal cells reveals novel patterns of gene expression during adipocyte differentiation. Stem Cell Res 16(3):725–734
14. van Vollenstee FA, Jackson C, Hoffmann D, Potgieter M, Durandt C, Pepper MS (2016) Human adipose derived mesenchymal stromal cells transduced with gfp lentiviral vectors: assessment of immunophenotype and differentiation capacity in vitro. Cytotechnology 68(5): 2049–2060
15. Durandt C, Dessels C, da Silva C, Murdoch C, Pepper MS (2019) The effect of early rounds of ex vivo expansion and cryopreservation on the adipogenic differentiation capacity of adipose-derived stromal/stem cells. Sci Rep 9(1): 15943
16. Dessels C, Pepper MS (2019) Reference gene expression in adipose-derived stromal cells undergoing adipogenic differentiation. Tissue Eng 25(6):353–366
17. Wolmarans E, Mellet J, Durandt C, Joubert F, Pepper MS (2021) Single-cell transcriptome analysis of human adipose-derived stromal cells identifies a contractile cell subpopulation. Stem Cells Int 2021:5595172
18. Dessels C, Ambele MA, Pepper MS (2019) The effect of medium supplementation and serial passaging on the transcriptome of human adipose-derived stromal cells expanded in vitro. Stem Cell Res Ther 10(1):253
19. Durandt C, Van Vollenstee FA, Dessels C, Kallmeyer K, De Villiers D, Murdoch C, Potgieter M, Pepper MS (2016) Novel flow cytometric approach for the detection of adipocyte sub-populations during adipogenesis. J Lipid Res 57(4):729–742
20. Dessels C, Potgieter M, Pepper MS (2016) Making the switch: alternatives to fetal bovine serum for adipose-derived stromal cell expansion. Front Cell Dev Biol 17(4):115–125. https://doi.org/10.3389/fcell.2016.00115
21. Dessels C, Durandt C, Pepper MS (2018) Comparison of human platelet lysate alternatives using expired and freshly isolated platelet concentrates for adipose-derived stromal cell expansion. Platelets 30:1–12
22. Orbay H, Tobita M, Mizuno H (2012) Mesenchymal stem cells isolated from adipose and

other tissues: basic biological properties and clinical applications. Stem Cells Int 2012: 461718. https://doi.org/10.1155/2012/461718

23. Hass R, Kasper C, Böhm S, Jacobs R (2011) Different populations and sources of human mesenchymal stem cells (MSC): a comparison of adult and neonatal tissue-derived MSC. Cell Commun Signal 9:12. https://doi.org/10.1186/1478-811X-9-12

24. Zhang QZ, Nguyen AL, Yu WH, Le AD (2012) Human oral mucosa and gingiva: a unique reservoir for mesenchymal stem cells. J Dent Res 91(11):1011–1018. https://doi.org/10.1177/0022034512461016

25. Burk J, Ribitsch I, Gittel C, Juelke H, Kasper C, Staszyk C, Brehm W (2013) Growth and differentiation characteristics of equine mesenchymal stromal cells derived from different sources. Vet J (London, England: 1997) 195(1):98–106. https://doi.org/10.1016/j.tvjl.2012.06.004

# Index



Michael S. Pepper and Melvin A. Ambele (eds.), *Adipogenesis: Methods and Protocols*, Methods in Molecular Biology, vol. 2938, https://doi.org/10.1007/978-1-0716-4607-6,

## G



## H



## I



## K



## L



## M



## N



## O



## P



## Q



## R



## S

MIX
Papier aus verantwortungsvollen Quellen
Paper from responsible sources
FSC® C105338

If you have any concerns about our products,
you can contact us on
**ProductSafety@springernature.com**

In case Publisher is established outside the EU,
the EU authorized representative is:
**Springer Nature Customer Service Center GmbH**
**Europaplatz 3, 69115 Heidelberg, Germany**

Printed by Libri Plureos GmbH
in Hamburg, Germany